Comprehensive Manuals of Surgical Specialties

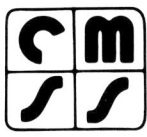

Richard H. Egdahl, editor

Manual of Aesthetic Surgery

Edited by
Jack C. Fisher, Jose Guerrerosantos, Matthew Gleason

Illustrated by Lena Lyons

Includes 134 illustrations, 81 in full color

Springer-Verlag
New York Berlin Heidelberg Tokyo

SERIES EDITOR

Richard H. Egdahl, M.D., Ph.D., Professor of Surgery, Boston University Medical Center, Boston, Massachusetts 02118 U.S.A.

EDITORS

Jack C. Fisher, M.D., Professor and Head, Division of Plastic Surgery, University of California, San Diego, Medical Center, San Diego, California 92103 U.S.A.

Jose Guerrerosantos, M.D., Director and Plastic Surgeon in Charge, The Jalisco Reconstructive Plastic Surgery Institute; Professor and Chairman of the Division of Plastic and Reconstructive Surgery, University of Guadalajara Medical College, Guadalajara, Mexico

Matthew Gleason, M.D., Clinical Professor of Surgery, Division of Plastic Surgery, Department of Surgery, University of California, San Diego Medical Center, 4103 Third Avenue, San Diego, California 92103 U.S.A.

Library of Congress Cataloging in Publication Data
Main entry under title:
Manual of aesthetic surgery.
  (Comprehensive manuals of surgical specialties)
  Bibliography: p.
  Includes index.
  1. Surgery, Plastic.   I. Fisher, Jack C., 1937–
II. Guerrerosantos, Jose.   III. Gleason, Matthew C.,
1926–   .   IV. Series.   [DNLM: 1. Surgery, Plastic.
WO 600 M2935]
RD119.M36   1985   617'.95   84-26831

© 1985 by Springer-Verlag New York Inc.

All rights reserved. No part of this book may be translated or reproduced in any form without written permission from Springer-Verlag, 175 Fifth Avenue, New York, New York 10010, U.S.A.

The use of general descriptive names, trade names, trademarks, etc., in this publication, even if the former are not especially identified, is not to be taken as a sign that such names, as understood by the Trade Marks and Merchandise Marks Act, may accordingly be used freely by anyone.

While the advice and information of this book is believed to be true and accurate at the date of going to press, neither the authors nor the editors nor the publisher can accept any legal responsibility for any errors or omissions that may be made. The publisher makes no warranty, express or implied, with respect to material contained herein.

Typeset by Kingsport Press, Kingsport, Tennessee.
Printed and bound by H. Stürtz AG, Würzburg, Federal Republic of Germany.
Printed in the Federal Republic of Germany.

9 8 7 6 5 4 3 2 1

ISBN 0-387-96045-7 Springer-Verlag New York Berlin Heidelberg Tokyo
ISBN 3-540-96045-7 Springer-Verlag Berlin Heidelberg New York Tokyo

Dedicated to our residents who will always force us to reexamine the validity of our convictions

Editor's Note

Comprehensive Manuals of Surgical Specialties is a series of surgical manuals designed to present current operative techniques and to explore various aspects of diagnosis and treatment. The series features a unique format with emphasis on large, detailed, full-color illustrations, schematic charts, and photographs to demonstrate integral steps in surgical procedures.

Each manual focuses on a specific region or topic and describes surgical anatomy, physiology, pathology, diagnosis, and operative treatment. Operative techniques and stratagems for dealing with surgically correctable disorders are described in detail. Illustrations are primarily depicted from the surgeon's viewpoint to enhance clarity and comprehension.

Other volumes in the series:

Published:

Manual of Endocrine Surgery (Second Edition)
Manual of Burns
Manual of Surgery of the Gallbladder, Bile Ducts, and Exocrine Pancreas
Manual of Gynecologic Surgery
Manual of Urologic Surgery
Manual of Lower Gastrointestinal Surgery
Manual of Vascular Surgery, Volume I
Manual of Cardiac Surgery, Volume I
Manual of Cardiac Surgery, Volume II
Manual of Liver Surgery
Manual of Ambulatory Surgery
Manual of Pulmonary Surgery
Manual of Soft Tissue Tumor Surgery
Manual of Vascular Access, Organ Donation, and Transplantation

In Preparation:

Manual of Vascular Surgery, Volume II
Manual of Orthopedic Surgery
Manual of Upper Gastrointestinal Surgery

Editor's Note

Manual of Trauma Surgery
Manual of Reconstructive Surgery
Manual of Sports Surgery
Manual of Gynecologic Surgery (Second Edition)

Richard H. Egdahl

Preface

Initially we asked Springer-Verlag why they thought the world needed another book about aesthetic surgery. They pointed to the popularity of the Comprehensive Manual of Surgical Specialties Series, suggesting that completeness required our contribution. We recalled the current masters of aesthetic surgery: Rees, Sheen, among others. Each had produced his own monograph—all of them established classics. What could we add? Furthermore none of us was recognized exclusively for aesthetic surgery achievements.

Nevertheless, each of us was committed to the challenge of teaching residents aesthetic surgery *during* their residency, not afterward as was done in the past. Furthermore, Dick Egdahl, Senior Editor and designer of CMSS, made clear to us the specific orientation of the manuals to residents-in-training. He won our support, as did Springer-Verlag, well known for their commitment to high-quality color illustrations.

We appreciate being asked by Dr. Egdahl to contribute to CMSS. We were not even offended by his original plan to embrace all of plastic surgery in one volume. He should have known better! The *Manual of Reconstructive Surgery* will follow this volume in 2 years. Defining its scope remains an unmet challenge.

Limiting the scope of *Manual of Aesthetic Surgery* has been an easier task. It is a sourcebook for beginning residents, not an encyclopedic reference. We have established in well-illustrated detail a single basic approach. Variations can be adopted as skill and judgment develop. The sequence of chapters progresses in approximately the same order that we assign responsibility to residents during their training: augmentation and abdominoplasty early on, followed by facelift and rhinoplasty. Essential facts are outlined in the order that residents must understand them as patients are selected and operative plans made. Complications and the characteristics of recovery come early, under the heading "What the Patient Needs to Know Before Surgery." Specific anatomic detail appears as "What the Surgeon Must Know." "Operative Design" is distinguished from "Operative Technique." Then come "Variations," i.e., alternative methods to get the job done properly. Finally "Issues" are considered, controversies for which the answers are not yet fully known. References are selective, sometimes annotated.

Preface

Our thanks go to Lena Lyons, who persevered with us during all the preoperative conferences, the many hours of observation and sketching (ably supervised by Fred Harwin), and the final critical review of each illustration for clarity and resident understanding. Her style involves showing it just the way it looks during the operation. We were doubly pleased when Lena, originally hired only to sketch, was selected by Springer to complete the coloring, a task she did so very well.

Jack C. Fisher

Jose Guerrerosantos

Matthew Gleason

Contents

Editor's Note vii
Preface ix
Contributors xv

1 Education of the Aesthetic Surgeon 1
Jack C. Fisher

2 Selecting Patients for Aesthetic Surgery 5
Sally Ann Greer and Matthew Gleason

Initial Screening Process 5
Additional Screening 6
Religious Considerations 7
How to Say No 8

3 Sedation for Aesthetic Surgery 9
Jack C. Fisher

The Importance of Sedation 9
Talk Is Cheap . . . and Effective 10
Preparation in Advance of Surgery 10
On the Day of Surgery 11
Choice of Drugs 11
Failure 11
Toward the End 12
Prior to Discharge 12
Later On . . . Check Yourself 12

4 Augmentation Mammaplasty 13
Jack C. Fisher and Ross Rudolph

Background 13
Indications 13
Potential Contraindications 14
What the Patient Needs to Know Before Surgery 15
What the Surgeon Must Know 15
Operative Design 16
Regional Anesthesia 16
Operative Technique 16
Variations 22
Issues 23

5 Breast Reduction/Elevation 25
Carson M. Lewis and Jack C. Fisher

Background 25
Indications 25
Contraindications 26
What the Patient Needs to Know Before Surgery 26
What the Surgeon Must Know 27
Operative Design 28
Anesthesia 29
Operative Technique 30
Variations 36
Issues 38

6 Abdominoplasty 39
Jose Guerrerosantos and Jack C. Fisher

Background 39
Indications 39
Potential Contraindications 39
What the Patient Needs to Know Before Surgery 40
What the Surgeon Must Know 40
Operative Planning 41
Anesthesia 41
Operative Technique 43
Variations 48

7 Blepharoplasty 51
Carson M. Lewis and Leonard W. Glass

Background 51
Indications 51

Contraindications 51
What the Patient Needs to Know Before Surgery 52
What the Surgeon Must Know 52
Operative Planning 53
Regional Anesthesia 54
Operative Techniques 54
Variations 56
Issues 57

8 Facelift 59
Matthew Gleason and Jose Guerrerosantos

Background 59
Indications 59
Contraindications 59
What the Patient Needs to Know Before Surgery 60
What the Surgeon Must Know 61
Operative Design 63
Anesthesia 64
Operative Technique 64
Variations 69
Issues 71

9 Necklift 75
Jose Guerrerosantos

Background 75
Indications 75
Contraindications 76
What the Patient Needs to Know Before Surgery 76
What the Surgeon Must Know 77
Operative Planning 79
Regional Anesthesia 79
Operative Technique 79
Variations 82
Issues 82

10 Forehead Lift 85
Matthew Gleason

Background 85
Indications 85
Contraindications 85
What the Patient Needs to Know Before Surgery 86
What the Surgeon Must Know 86
Operative Design 88
Anesthesia 88

Operative Technique 89
Variations 95
Issues 96

11 Rhinoplasty 99
Leonard W. Glass and Thomas Donovan

Background 99
Indications 99
Potential Contraindications 100
What the Patient Needs to Know Before Surgery 100
What the Surgeon Must Know 101
Operative Planning 102
Regional Anesthesia 103
Operative Technique 106
Variations 111
Issues 112

12 Dermabrasion, Chemical Peel, and Collagen Injection 113
David H. Frank and Leonard W. Glass

Dermabrasion 113
  Indications 113
  Contraindications 114
  What the Patient Needs to Know Before the Procedure 114
  Regional Anesthesia 114
  Technique 115
Chemical Peel 115
  Indications 115
  Contraindications 116
  What the Patient Needs to Know Before the Procedure 116
  What the Surgeon Needs to Know 116
  Regional Anesthesia 117
  Technique 117
Collagen Injection 118
  Indications 118
  Contraindications 119
  What the Patient Needs to Know Before the Procedure 119
  What the Surgeon Must Know 120
  Technique 121
  Variations 121

Index 123

Contributors

Thomas L. Donovan, M.D., Assistant Clinical Professor of Surgery, Division of Plastic Surgery, Department of Surgery, University of California, San Diego, Medical Center, San Diego, California

Jack C. Fisher, M.D., Professor and Head, Division of Plastic Surgery, Department of Surgery, University of California, San Diego, Medical Center, San Diego, California

David H. Frank, M.D., Associate Professor of Surgery, Division of Plastic Surgery, Department of Surgery, University of California, San Diego, Medical Center, San Diego, California

Leonard W. Glass, M.D., Clinical Professor of Surgery, Division of Plastic Surgery, Department of Surgery, University of California, San Diego, Medical Center, San Diego, California

Matthew Gleason, M.D., Clinical Professor of Surgery, Division of Plastic Surgery, Department of Surgery, University of California, San Diego, Medical Center, San Diego, California

Sally Ann Greer, Ph.D., Clinical Psychologist, Private Practice; Consultant to U.S. Department of State, Washington, D.C.

Jose Guerrerosantos, M.D., Director and Plastic Surgeon in Charge, The Jalisco Reconstructive Plastic Surgery Institute; Professor and Chairman of the Division of Plastic and Reconstructive Surgery, University of Guadalajara Medical College, Guadalajara, Mexico

Carson M. Lewis, M.D., Assistant Clinical Professor of Surgery, Division of Plastic Surgery, Department of Surgery, University of California, San Diego, Medical Center, San Diego, California

Ross Rudolph, M.D., Associate Clinical Professor of Surgery, Division of Plastic Surgery, Department of Surgery, University of California, San Diego, Medical Center, San Diego, California

Education of the Aesthetic Surgeon

Jack C. Fisher

A brief look at the history of plastic surgery shows that the estrangement of aesthetic surgery from mainstream medical practice is a longstanding and continuing phenomenon. The traditional priorities of medical science have always been assigned to the gravely ill, not to the physically deformed. Furthermore, surgeons who had applied their skills to "superficial" issues such as appearance endured the scorn of their professional colleagues.

After the two great wars, some respectability for plastic surgeons was established because correction of wartime injuries became a social imperative. Today, relative political stability and economic prosperity have produced increasing demand for aesthetic surgery. At the same time, nonmilitary indications for reconstructive surgery have not kept pace with the rate at which we are training new plastic surgeons. Add to this modern-day price competitive forces in health care financing that seek to limit socioeconomically valid indications for reconstructive surgery and it is easy to see why plastic surgery once again assumes a "superficial" character in the eyes of practicing physicians.

Medical schools have not traditionally assigned high priority to recruitment of academic plastic surgeons whose remunerative appetites can exceed what deans are willing to pay. As a result, aesthetic surgery is either removed from a medical student's clinical exposure or its practice is absorbed into otolaryngologic, sometimes even dermatologic, services. Even when plastic surgeons are represented on a medical school faculty, the teaching of aesthetic surgery may be assigned low priority. A resident's clinical experience usually parallels the interests of his program director.

In the past, aesthetic surgical skills were considered privileged information and withheld from discussion. Jacques Joseph demanded a significant fee from students admitted to his operating room. Even then, certain technical maneuvers were withheld from view. Joseph realized the importance of preserving his market by limiting competition. If he were alive today, he would probably consider foolish the predicament we have created by training plastic surgeons in excess of market demand.

Contributors to this Manual can recall their own mentors going to a hospital remote from the residency training site to practice their aesthetic surgery. Or we can remember serving only an assisting role in aesthetic surgery during residency, learning on our own during the early years of practice. Trial-and-error is certainly not the preferred method for learning surgery;

yet this is the way many surgeons have learned how to select patients, how to say no, how to collect aesthetic fees in advance, how to develop a range of techniques to meet individual patient need rather than to perfect a single method, how to manipulate tissue within narrow margins of error, how to provide the necessary patient encouragement throughout the recovery period, how to deal with patient dissatisfaction, and how to respond sensibly to litigation.

This volume outlines the essential curriculum for aesthetic surgery instruction, best completed during the residency, not afterwards. No longer should we permit graduation from an accredited training program without ensuring adequate opportunity to learn every challenge of aesthetic practice. We are not the only specialty with expressed interests in this field. Hospital credential committees are at present adapting to the excess number of surgeons by asking for and expecting to see documentation of operative experience during residency.

I know program directors who practice a bold and imaginative style of reconstructive surgery. "There is nothing to aesthetic surgery," they declare. Yet aesthetic surgery can be the Achilles heel of the new surgeon in practice. Although technically capable, he might not deal comfortably with the high expectations of the aesthetic patient. From experience it is my belief that aesthetic surgery is perhaps the greatest teaching challenge in a residency program curriculum; the margins for error are so narrow, the demands of the patient so great, and the need for surgeon sensitivity is even greater.

This Manual represents an outgrowth of the experience of two training programs, one in San Diego, the other in Guadalajara. Our commitment has been to make certain that residents receive both reconstructive and aesthetic surgery experience during their training. We have learned the following lessons:

1. Residents must be given access to a population of patients desirous of aesthetic surgery at a reduced fee on a teaching service. Some of these patients would not have sought surgery without fee reduction whereas others ultimately might have found a private surgeon. A teaching service for aesthetic surgery is therefore in competition with community plastic surgeons and also with academic surgeons who practice aesthetic surgery. Resident opportunity in aesthetic surgery should therefore be considered a gift from the community of plastic surgeons. In return, the training program owes to its nearby colleagues a limit on reduced-fee surgery, perhaps also a limit on the number of residents trained in that community.

2. Reduced-fee aesthetic surgery must be an open contractual arrangement with full disclosure. We make clear to patients that residents will serve as the principal surgeons under the guidance and supervision of a fully qualified plastic surgeon.

3. A careful distinction should be made between a resident in postgraduate surgical training and an intern or junior level trainee. Only the senior resident is permitted opportunity for aesthetic practice. Patients might otherwise conclude that their surgery will be done by an inexperienced hand.

4. Prospective patients should always meet the senior resident well in advance; a doctor–patient relationship is established before a surgical commitment is made.

5. Some patients are comfortable with this arrangement whereas others are not. A choice is offered but coercion is never used. Surgery by an attending surgeon is always an alternative.

6. A qualified plastic surgeon should be present for supervision of all aesthetic surgery performed by residents.

7. Fee arrangements vary from one institution to another. In ours, the patient must meet the costs of facility use. Residents are therefore stimulated to limit those costs, to use operating time efficiently. In addition, a modest "training fee" is charged for professional supervision. These funds are used to support cost of residency training but may not be used to supplement resident salaries.

8. Reduced-fee aesthetic surgery patients must pay in advance just as private patients do.

9. Residents participate in the patient selection process, the surgery, and the recovery. In the event of complications or dissatisfaction, residents deal with these problems as well, also under experienced supervision.

10. Most gratifying is our observation that residents experience growth of their aesthetic practice during residency; new patients come via referral from satisfied patients just as will be true later when their own practice develops. Furthermore, the nature and frequency of complaints or complications is no different than it is for the full-time or voluntary faculty.

Additional Reading

Rogers BO. The development of aesthetic surgery: A history. Aesth Plast Surg 1:3–24, 1976.

Rees TD. Aesthetic Plastic Surgery. Saunders, Philadelphia, 1980.

Selecting Patients for Aesthetic Surgery

Sally Ann Greer and Matthew Gleason

The same attention must be devoted to learning how to select patients for aesthetic surgery as is devoted to perfecting surgical technique. This principle may not be easily accepted by the resident-in-training but it will be embraced by experienced surgeons who remain challenged by the patient selection process.

People who seek aesthetic surgery are not typical of the general population; yet studies have shown them to be more stable than generally assumed by most physicians. The real challenge of aesthetic surgery involves matching technical possibility with patient desire. "*All* aesthetic surgery patients have unreasonable expectations," declared one experienced and candid plastic surgeon. His intention was to convey the belief that the surgeon tries to select those whom he hopes to satisfy and avoid those he fears he cannot please.

Initial Screening Process

During the initial interview, the surgeon must be alert for signals that indicate potentials for success or failure. Some important questions are: Who? What? When? Why?

Who?

Who referred the patient, or how did the patient select you? Often, a satisfied patient will be the source of referral. If the patient is referred by another physician, opportunity exists to discuss the patient with that colleague. The patient's physical and mental stability can be discussed. Insights can be shared regarding the patient's motivation, keeping in mind that physicians in other fields are sometimes not qualified to analyze or judge a patient's motivation for aesthetic surgery.

If a patient refuses to identify the source of referral, suspect prior unsatisfactory surgery or consultation. There is nothing wrong in seeking more than one opinion; however, problem patients can carry this principle to extremes.

Some who seek your counsel will describe and demonstrate prior surgery that you might consider beneath your standard. Do not accept all of these patients; you will surely not satisfy them all! A small percentage can be called "insatiable," meaning that neither you nor any surgeon will likely meet that patient's needs.

What?

What does the patient want? Ask your patient to define the problem before you do. Ask that priorities be established. "If I could correct only one problem, which would that be?" Next priority? Next?

Ask also what brings the patient to your office now. Are there outside forces at work? A marital partner? A lost job opportunity? Pressure from a friend? A relative? This is a time when external motivating forces, if any, can be distinguished from the internal needs of the patient.

The problem patient cannot easily define a problem. Nonspecific requests such as "Just fix my nose" are insufficient for reasonable surgical planning. Alteration of an ethnic or parental identity may not be biologically possible.

When?

Ask when the patient first began to consider surgery. Then ask when he or she wants to have surgery scheduled.

Ideal patients will describe a longstanding desire for surgery, and they are willing to plan weeks and months ahead. The least desirable patient thought of the procedure yesterday and wants it done tomorrow! Impulsive patients usually experience displeasure following a surgeon's most extraordinary efforts on their behalf.

Why?

Further into the conversation, ask why. This will require patient analysis, insight, and perhaps speculation. Some will have a clear explanation, others will not. There are no totally correct answers to this question but there are a few wrong answers:

Do they expect surgery to change their opportunities in life? Will surgery gain them a job? Will intimate relationships evolve when they have escaped capture in the past? Does the image of a celebrity yield anticipation of the excitement of living that individual's coveted existence? Obviously these are all unrealistic expectations beyond possibility of attainment through surgery.

Studies show that following surgery, improvements in self-esteem can yield perceptions of improved quality of life, but these are subtle changes, not dramatic life transformations.

Additional Screening

The initial screening interview allows the surgeon to construct a composite of the patient's background, needs, expectations, and motivation.

Additional goals, perhaps not achievable until the second consultation, include informing patients of the exact nature of surgery, identifying specific contraindications, or determining any factors that alert the surgeon to possible trouble ahead.

A fully informed patient should not be surprised by any event associated with surgery. Use of terminology understandable to the patient is essential. Matching goals with reality depends on both the surgeon and the perception of the patient once the facts are explained.

Situational contraindications may be temporary, e.g., unstable medical or emotional status, recent stress such as personal or family illness, death of a loved one, or a divorce. Never forget that surgery, all surgery, is a stress, not just a physiologic stress during the event, but also an emotional stress throughout the period of healing. Patients should be asked to handle only one major stress at a time.

Always take into account the specific mental disorders that can lead to trouble. Preexisting depression, a common disorder, must be spotted. If under proper treatment, then surgery may not be contraindicated. Always warn these patients that temporary reactive depression is commonplace following surgery. Perhaps a psychiatrist should be called upon for supportive medication during the recovery period.

The neurotic, psychotic, and sociopath (character disorder) are labels for maladaptive behavior patterns. Any apparent display of these behaviors should trigger in the surgeon an intuitive sense that trouble lies ahead.

The psychotic has lost appropriate linkage between feeling, objects, and appearances. This patient's hold on reality is tenuous. The "walking psychotics," if they can call for an appointment and arrive on time, may not always demonstrate confusion, disorientation, or overt lack of reality testing. But they will usually fail to define specific needs or expectations. Neither are they capable of coordinating a decision for surgery with the rest of their lives.

The more obvious psychotics are likely to display excessive suspiciousness or fear of persecution. Some psychotic individuals may be legitimate candidates for aesthetic surgery. Nevertheless, the plastic surgeon cannot proceed without the recommendation and continuing support of a psychiatrist.

Neurotic patients may or may not display anxiety or excessive worry. They often feel overly responsible for the events in their lives or the lives of others. Not every patient displaying neurotic behavior should be refused aesthetic surgery.

Patients with character disorders deserve prompt recognition by the plastic surgeon, especially the manipulative patient and the infantile/narcissistic patient. Common to both are avoidance of decision-making or responsibility. These patients experience profound interpersonal communication gaps and persistently seek the missing element in their lives. Surgery is often sought as a vehicle to achieve these ends, but not often with success!

Manipulative patients establish a strong need for service, but only at their convenience, never the surgeon's. They initially appear confident, even organized. They overuse the pronoun "I." "I want," "I need," "I know you can do it for me." These patients are superficially likeable, and quite often flatter the surgeon's skill, e.g., "I have heard all about you and I'm certain you are the only one who can solve my problem."

Difficulties with payment often arise with these patients. The manipulative patient will convince your secretary to postpone request for payment until the first postoperative visit, which is always a mistake. Once surgery is past, nothing is satisfactory because of course nothing has ever been satisfactory for these patients.

Infantile/narcissistic patients demonstrate total belief in and trust of the surgeon; this is how they relieve themselves of responsibility for their actions. These patients always appeal to the surgeon's greater wisdom and experience, saying: "You decide what I need . . ." "I know you will make all of the best decisions." Narcissistic patients are also likeable but difficult nonetheless.

Plastic surgeons who covet adoration are unusually vulnerable to patients with character disorders. But whenever the surgeon takes responsibility for their welfare, he will also be held accountable for failing to solve their problems.

Religious Considerations

Often overlooked are some very subtle but specific religious barriers to patient acceptance of aesthetic surgery.

The use of surgery for the improvement of appearance can be considered forbidden according to individual interpretation of existing religious doctrine. Be alert to the following sectarian positions that may result in patient ambivalence or conflict, not only prior to surgery but also afterwards.

Roman Catholics adhere to the "principle of totality." This doctrine specifies that the parts of the body are ordained to the good of the whole person. A patient therefore ought not to alter the body to enhance seductiveness, gratify vanity, harm a normal function, or to escape justice. Alteration of the body is acceptable whenever the intention is moral and when the patient will not be exposed to risk.

Your Roman Catholic patient may not express these concerns willingly but may nevertheless seek inward resolution of these issues. For anticipated breast augmentation or reduction, preservation of breast function may be of paramount concern.

The Protestant, especially the fundamental Protestant, maintains grave concerns about vanity and seductiveness. Issues influencing selfishness or pride may also lead to conflict. These patients will seek to justify their decision based on the influence their improved self-esteem might have on their families or loved ones.

The conservative Jewish view of surgical alteration is based on the belief that the body is not owned by the individual. Therefore aesthetic surgery may be contraindicated whenever life is endangered, if the body is mutilated, or if postsurgical changes will be viewed as an attack on divine plan. A favorable view of surgery depends on the procedure alleviating a problem that prevents marriage, makes for unhappiness in an existing marriage, or prevents an individual from playing a constructive role in society.

Only rarely will patients express their religious concerns to their surgeon. What will be important is not what the surgeon says but rather what the patient subsequently believes or works out internally. Nevertheless, bring this subject up if you suspect conflicts. Urge patients to seek the advice of clergy. Meanwhile, postpone surgery.

How to Say No

Many plastic surgeons would stay out of trouble if they could more easily say no. Denying a patient surgery is not an easy task. You must also decide whether you should reject a patient altogether or merely postpone a decision.

I know surgeons who can easily refuse to do surgery and even suggest that the patient not ever return. This relieves both the surgeon and front office staff of any further waste of time. But the "cold turkey" approach can also stimulate hostility and generate ill-will in the very community from which in time will come future patients.

Postponement is the other approach. Tell the patient that surgery is not appropriate at this time. Also define the conditions for future reconsideration of surgery, psychiatric or psychologic consultation, etc. Not often will patients accept referral to a behavioral discipline; those who do may appreciate your willingness to keep surgery a possible option after emotional problems are resolved.

Irrespective of the behavioral diagnosis, hope is a force not to be treated callously or abandoned. Therefore retain an option of surgery if it is remotely feasible. In the meantime offer worthwhile justification for delay, including when appropriate referral for counseling.

Additional Reading

Goin JM and Goin MK. Changing the Body. Williams & Wilkins, Baltimore, 1981.

Sedation for Aesthetic Surgery

3

Jack C. Fisher

In many regions of the world, general anesthesia is used routinely for aesthetic surgery, making sedation a less important step. In the future, increasing costs of surgery will very likely stimulate more frequent use of local anesthesia. In the United States, where hospital costs are prohibitive, patients requesting elective surgery will seek surgeons willing to use sedation and local anesthesia in preference to general anesthesia, usually in an office operating facility.

The Importance of Sedation

The following vignette illustrates just how important sedation can be:

> The patient was prompt but the door was locked! She paced 1 minute, 2, then 10. The nurse arrived, unlocked the door, and asked her to be seated. Soon the nurse reappeared and said the patient's chart was missing. The patient wondered if she had come the wrong day but just then an assistant resident arrived, grumbled about the missing workup, and set about repeating the examination. He would have to draw blood again as well . . . the lab results were also missing. The patient wondered if she would be asked to pay twice for her blood tests.
>
> The phone rang. Her surgeon's office was on the phone; had she remembered her check? The nurse seemed to glare. Yes she had; it was in her purse, now safe in her locker. She would have to go and get it now; those were the secretary's orders!
>
> Blood sample redrawn, the nurse announced that an IV would soon be started. "Why not accomplish both goals with one needle stick?" the patient asked but her query went unanswered. Perhaps she had been unheard; someone had turned on a radio . . . country/western, rather loud. She hated western music but no one had asked her opinion.
>
> Her surgeon was not present. She asked why and the nurse replied, "He is often late. He keeps us waiting; then he rushes."
>
> "I hope he doesn't rush with me!" exclaimed the patient as she felt a rising panic within.
>
> She was moved into an icy cold operating room; wires were attached to her shoulders. She wondered why? As the nurse began to wash her breasts, she noticed a stranger at the scrub sink staring into the room.

At last her surgeon appeared in the doorway, waved hello and said, "Good morning, how are you doing?"

"Fine," said the patient.

"Her blood pressure is a little high, Doctor," said the nurse."

"What am I doing here?" wondered the patient to herself.

Does this sound exaggerated? Not at all! I have seen something like this happen in a teaching hospital setting, more than once I'm sorry to say.

What was missing? Powerful sedatives? Yes indeed, but words were also missing, preferably words spoken by the patient's surgeon as he brought her to a state of confident calm.

Talk Is Cheap . . . and Effective

The power of words as a preoperative sedative was effectively demonstrated in a controlled study of patients admitted for surgery. One group was visited by an anesthesiologist before surgery. Informative conversation was substituted for sedatives. A second group received conversation and barbiturate. The third group received barbiturate but no conversation.

The results were striking. Patients receiving only sedative drugs fared least well, required more anesthetic agent during surgery, and demanded more analgesia following surgery. Those benefitting from conversation before surgery did better, requiring less anesthetic agent and less pain medication afterward. Barbiturate offered only modest advantage in the group receiving both drug and conversation.

Preparation in Advance of Surgery

Your goal is a fully informed and confident patient, who is as calm as personality and neurophysiology will permit. Preparation begins long before surgery, perhaps before you become involved. At the moment of initial contact, your hospital or office staff can significantly influence your patient's attitude toward surgery.

Preparation continues during your first interview and throughout all subsequent conversations prior to surgery. I discuss a procedure at least twice before committing myself. I learn a great deal more about my patient at the second meeting. Distribution of fact sheets and information booklets also serves to develop patient confidence.

Complete all financial transactions in advance of the surgery day. The rule on our service, learned the hard way, is *payment in hand 1 week in advance of surgery* in order to reserve operating time. This is an especially important policy for teaching patients whose resources may be limited; they also sometimes engage in wishful thinking up until the moment payment is due, at which time fiscal reality takes hold and the patient either cancels or fails to show.

Residents-in-training are characteristically embarrassed to announce a payment-in-advance policy; yet we insist they do it. Office staff can reinforce but never substitute for a surgeon discussing fees directly with the patient.

If payment is not in hand 1 week ahead, surgery is cancelled but patients are gently offered opportunity to book in the future. Using this policy, residents learn quickly if the patient is sincere. Valuable operating time will not be lost. Financial issues are *never* handled on the day of surgery, a time when anxiety runs high.

On the Day of Surgery

All patients arrive with apprehension, latent anxiety, and a need to witness confirmation of all that has been told them. A nurse cannot substitute for the surgeon at this critical moment. I recommend that *you* be present, start the IV yourself, and most important, talk your patient into a confident mood. Do *not* complain about absent or deficient equipment. This is not a time for doctor–nurse power plays. This is a time to convince your patient that everything is happening the way you planned it (even if it isn't).

Background noise should be minimized. If music is available in the operating room, request your patient's permission and preference. Limit the number of people who enter the operating room, especially for breast surgery; and introduce each one; permit no one to stare into the room from the scrub area. Drape a hand towel over windows if necessary.

Choice of Drugs

Drugs are an individual matter and space does not permit a pharmacologic review. A few principles are listed:

1. Do not think you can accomplish all your goals with a single drug. You must provide three distinct effects: (a) sedation, (b) analgesia, and (c) relaxation. Few drugs are effective for more than one purpose.
2. Sedation comes first, and takes the longest to develop. Pentobarbital (Nembutal) is an excellent choice. A good technique is to give an oral dose at the moment of arrival, perhaps an hour before surgery. Alternatively, give all drugs by vein after the IV is started. Intramuscular administration is unnecessarily painful. Use a conservative sedative dose for the elderly patient.
3. Analgesia is best achieved with a narcotic. Ask your patient for a history of nausea following prior administration; govern your choice accordingly. Do not give so much narcotic that you have little room to administer small increments during the procedure.
4. Give your relaxant (e.g., diazepam (Valium)) immediately prior to administering local anesthesia. These are fast-acting and short-lived drugs. You want maximum effect at the moment of greatest discomfort, when local anesthesia is injected. Never rely on relaxants alone.
5. You will need higher doses of one or more of these drug categories if your patient has taken any one of them chronically in the past.
6. Alternate small doses of analgesic and relaxant throughout surgery. Supplementary barbiturates do not provide much advantage and can yield a dissociated and uncooperative patient.
7. Finally, do not forget conversation! I am convinced that my patients require less drug because I talk to them throughout surgery, anticipating each new major movement or source of discomfort, offering good news when appropriate ("We're more than halfway done now").

Failure

No matter how thorough your efforts, you will fail from time to time. When faced with a patient out-of-control, a rising diastolic blood pressure, or increased bleeding, back off; call for an anesthetist.

Note that patients of certain ethnic backgrounds (e.g., Mediterranean, Middle Eastern) are less appropriate for surgical procedures under regional anesthesia. It is not that they are weaker; they are merely accustomed to demonstrating their emotions. It is a lifelong trait you will not change. Northern Europeans can hide their feelings and are therefore more suited to regional anesthesia.

Toward the End

Do not keep giving narcotic as the procedure draws to an end. You will soon terminate your stimulation. The cumulative administration of drug may result in heavy sedation, and perhaps respiratory depression. More often than not, pain at the end of the procedure can be handled with supplementary local anesthesia (e.g., near the wound edges) rather than supplementary analgesia.

Prior to Discharge

Observe patients 1–3 h in the office or in outpatient center recovery before discharge. Anticipate for family members that the patient will sleep at home. However, they must remain easily arousable. Make certain an intelligent responsible friend or family member is present through the night.

Later On . . . Check Yourself

When you're learning, make certain you ask your patient during the postoperative period whether pain was a problem. If so, when? How bad? How could I have alleviated it?

You will be surprised what you learn. It does no good for patients to keep their impressions hidden. Your patient will tell her friends whether or not you were painful, so you had best know also. How else will you know if there is room for improvement?

Your goal is for your pleased patient to refer her friends because you were considerate, gentle, and knew what you were doing. These impressions are often created independent of the technical act of surgery.

Additional Reading

Egbert LD, Battit GE, Turndorf H, and Beecher HK. The value of the preoperative visit by an anesthetist. JAMA 185:553–555, 1963.

Augmentation Mammaplasty

4

Jack C. Fisher and Ross Rudolph

Background

Public demand for surgical enlargement of the breasts is not a recent derivative of the "Playboy Philosophy." Anthropologists tell us that throughout history and in numerous cultures, fascination with body form has been evident, particularly with respect to mammary proportion.

Credit is usually given to Czerny for the first augmentation mammaplasty. In 1895, he successfully transplanted a lipoma from the back to fill a defect resulting from removal of a benign breast adenoma. Lexer continued to popularize fat transplantation for breast enlargement early in this century. During and after World War II, Berson and Peer documented a rapid rate of fat resorption and advocated dermal fat grafts based on the hope that prompt vascularization of a dermal surface would impede fat atrophy.

A number of local flaps were suggested at various times, but each was associated with more scarring than was considered desirable by patients or their surgeons.

The era of implantable alloplastic materials began in 1899 when Gersuny described injection of paraffin. Other substances used for breast enlargement prior to silicone included vegetable oil, lanolin, beeswax, ivory, glass, Ivalon,® polethylene, and Etheron.® Silicone rubber was a development of the rapid industrialization following World War II. Medical application began after 1950. At the Third International Congress for Plastic and Reconstructive Surgery held in Washington, D.C. in 1963, Cronin and Gerow initially reported use of a silicone gel implantable breast prosthesis developed in cooperation with Dow Corning Corporation between 1960 and 1962, and first implanted in 1962.

The rest is modern history.

Indications

1. Developmental
   Symmetric hypoplasia (see Fig. 4–1)
   Asymmetric hypoplasia (sometimes associated with pectus aplasia (e.g., Poland's syndrome)
2. Traumatic
   Postburn deformity
   Postirradiation hypoplasia

3. Malignant
   Postmastectomy deformity
   Premalignancy leading to subcutaneous mastectomy
4. Degenerative
   Postpartum atrophy
5. Occupational (e.g., entertainer)

The vast majority of women seeking augmentation have symmetric hypoplasia, married patients outnumber unmarried, and their expectations are as a rule reasonable.

Potential Contraindications

1. Presence of a dominant external motive, e.g., pressure from a boyfriend or a dissatisfied husband.
2. Expectations beyond reality (e.g., cannot accept presence of scars, wanting to appear identical to an image in a photograph, etc.)

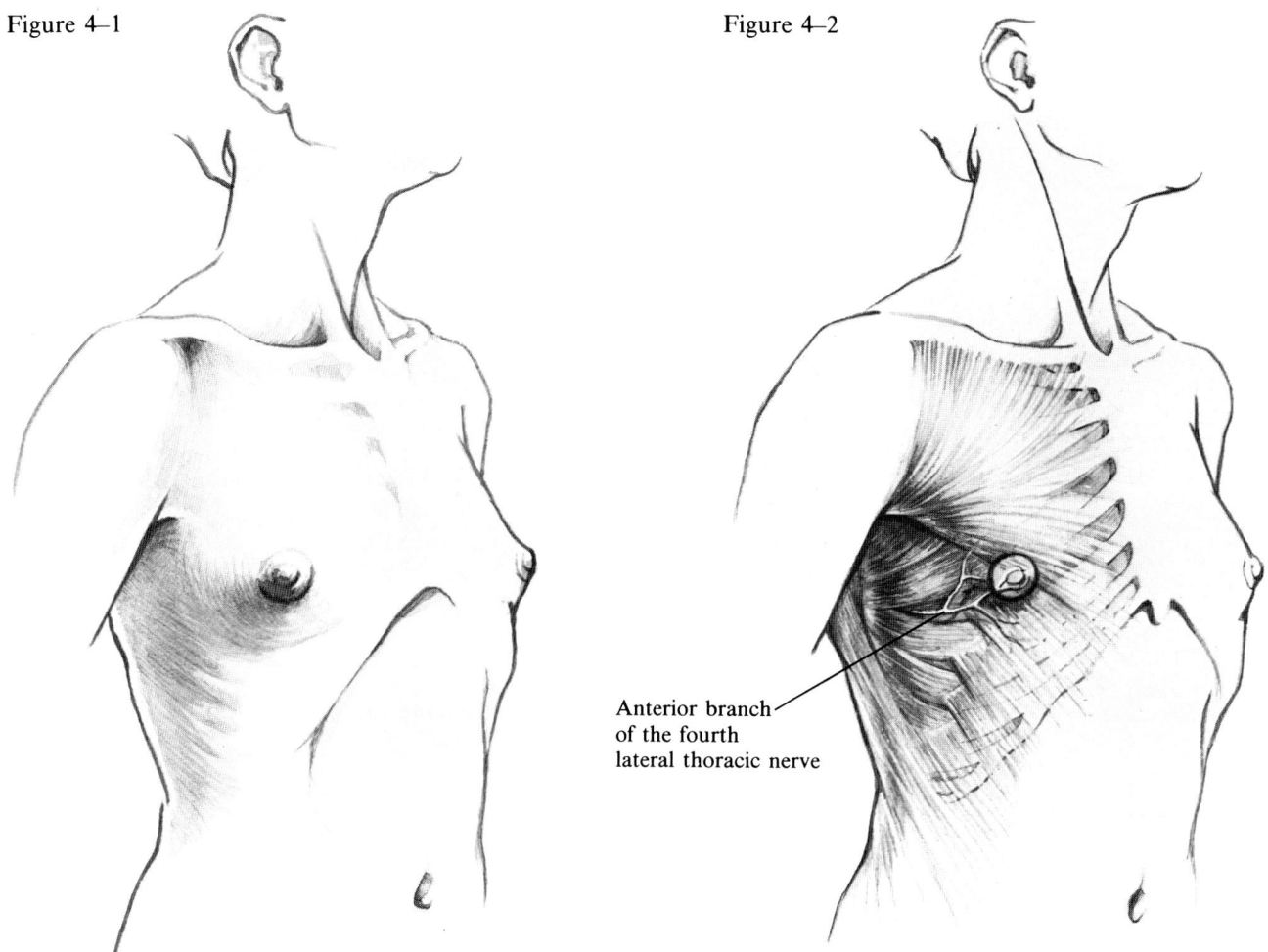

Figure 4–1

Figure 4–2

Anterior branch of the fourth lateral thoracic nerve

3. Unwillingness to accept risk of potential complications (e.g., breast firmness, diminished nipple sensitivity)
4. Poor financial planning (a surgeon does his patient no favor if the procedure or its complications are not affordable.)
5. Immature patient
6. Ptosis (nipple below inframammary fold)

Other relative contraindications include:

7. Genetic predisposition to hypertrophic scars
8. Painful fibrocystic disease
9. Previous silicone injections
10. "Tubular" areola or nipples
11. Emotional instability
12. Inability of prior surgeons to achieve satisfaction
13. Thick inelastic skin (older nullipara).

What the Patient Needs to Know Before Surgery

1. Site of incision: inframammary vs. periareolar
2. Nature of implant including possibility of a manufacturing defect.
3. Likelihood of postoperative breast firmness (a majority of patients experience breasts firmer than they would prefer; 10% develop firmness that is a problem, e.g., pain or distortion requiring secondary surgery).
4. Frequency of hematoma (fewer than 5%), infection (fewer than 2%), and extrusion (fewer than 1%). There is probably no such thing as "rejection."
5. Frequency of diminished nipple sensitivity (30% temporary, rare case of permanent anesthesia.
6. Effect on lactation (may be temporarily stimulated after surgery).
7. Absence of a reported malignancy arising from implanted silicone (as of this writing).
8. Menstrual cycle may be temporarily interrupted following surgery.
9. Final breast size is achieved 6 weeks following surgery (after swelling recedes).
10. Cleavage is not always possible.
11. Breast self-examination capability is not hindered.
12. Presence of an implant does not prevent accurate mammographic examination.

What the Surgeon Must Know

Normal but hypoplastic breasts may differ in size. Asymmetry of 10–15% is not unusual but should be noted prior to surgery. The nipple of the nonptotic breast rests between the fourth and fifth interspace, well above the inframammary fold. The breast is an organ of the skin, not of the chest wall. Therefore, the dissection plane between the breast and the pectoralis fascia (also beneath the pectoralis) is relatively avascular.

The anterior branch of the fourth lateral thoracic nerve is responsible for innervation of the nipple (see Fig. 4–2) and must not be injured during lateral dissection of the implant pocket. This nerve may be visualized as it passes through the serratus anterior muscle and enters the breast.

Operative Design

1. Placement of incision: For most surgeons, this means an inframammary incision (see Issues for discussion of periareolar site). The incision is placed slightly above the inframammary fold so that the scar will rest on the augmented breast and be less visible when brief garments are worn. Many prefer to mark the incision site in advance with the patient sitting (see Figs. 4–3 and 4–4). Patients will be displeased if the incisions are not symmetric. The incision averages 5 cm in length, $\frac{2}{3}$ medial to midline and $\frac{1}{3}$ lateral.
2. An important consideration is the extent of pocket dissection. There must be sufficient space to accommodate the implant with room to spare. The pocket begins at the incision, extends medially to the sternal border although not to midline, superiorly to within 2–3 cm of the clavicle, laterally to the extent of the existing breast (avoiding injury to the nerve of the nipple), and 1–2 cm inferior to the incision. Patients with a wide thorax will accept larger implants than those with a narrow chest.

Regional Anesthesia

Use 0.50% xylocaine with 1:2000,000 epinephrine. Maximum bilateral dose to avoid toxicity will be 100 cc in the average individual. First, infiltrate the previously marked incision site. Raise a linear wheel within the dermis, then extend deeper into the subcutaneous layer. Change to a No. 25 spinal needle and administer drug within the plane to be dissected—above the muscle, but beneath the breast. Some prefer to make an incision before continuing their field block, feeling they can direct the longer needle through the open incision better than they can percutaneously. Avoid rough traction on the breast. The patient is often both apprehensive and sensitive at this stage. Severe breast traction can be annoying as well as distort the passage of the needle.

One variation is intercostal block. Some prefer to block the second through fifth nerves, but risk of pneumothorax is significant.

Operative Technique

1. A careful prep and drape are essential because a foreign body is being used. Use of a preoperative antibiotic is habitual for some surgeons, never used by others.
2. The side first anesthetized is first dissected. Extend incision through subcutaneous incision to the serratus fascia, and insert a double hook into the glandular tissue visible beneath the upper incision border. Dissect superiorly with a knife or Metzenbaum® scissors until the pink border of the pectoralis major is encountered (Fig. 4–5). You will find it faster medially. It is easy for the novice to slip beneath the pectoralis.
3. Continue dissecting superior to the pectoralis fasica. If you see individual muscle fibers, you are one layer too deep. Finger dissection is easiest beginning 2 cm superior to pectoralis edge but only when superficial to the pectoralis fasic (Fig. 4–6).
4. Tell the patient when you convert to finger dissection. Give additional sedation and anesthesia when necessary. Some patients are sensitive to digital dissection. If so, back off, insert a lighted retractor, and continue dissection with extra long scissors under direct view. Avoid patient discomfort even if it takes a little longer. She will refer her friends to you only if she can say you were gentle!

Operative Technique

Figure 4–3

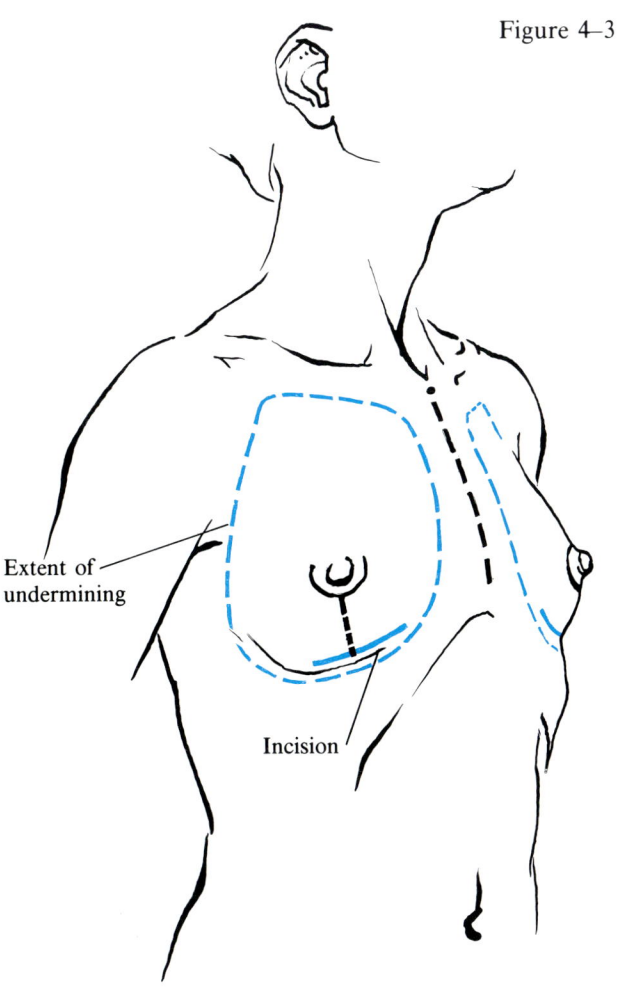

Extent of undermining

Incision

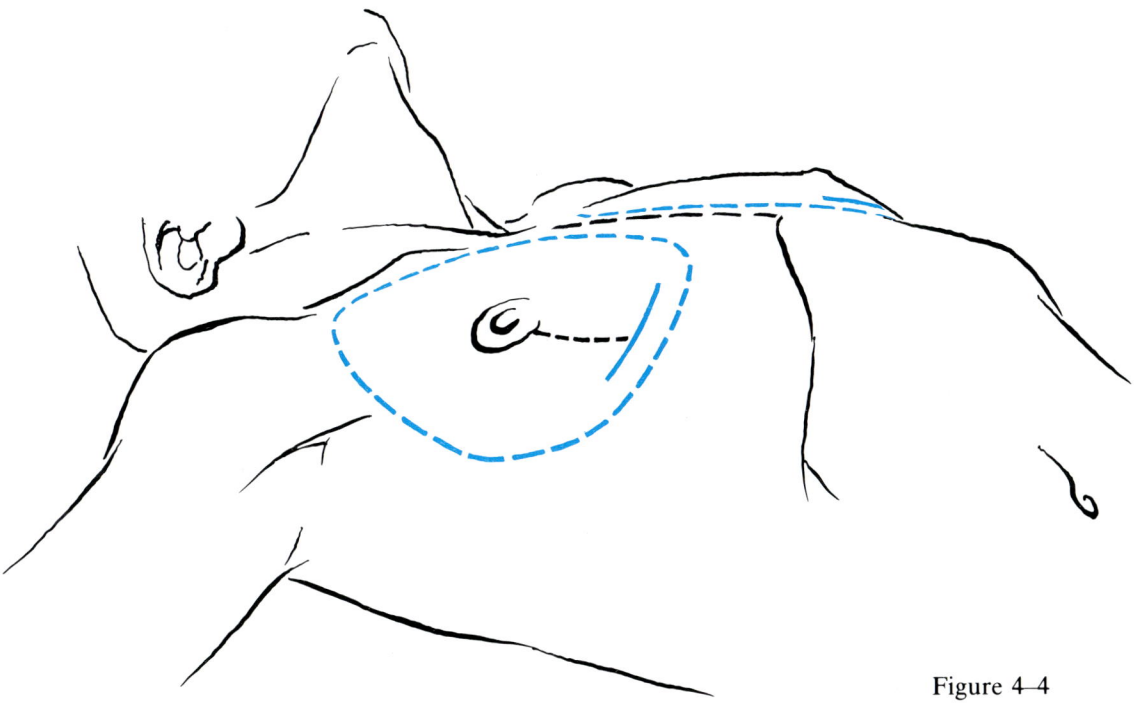

Figure 4–4

Augmentation Mammaplasty

Figure 4–5

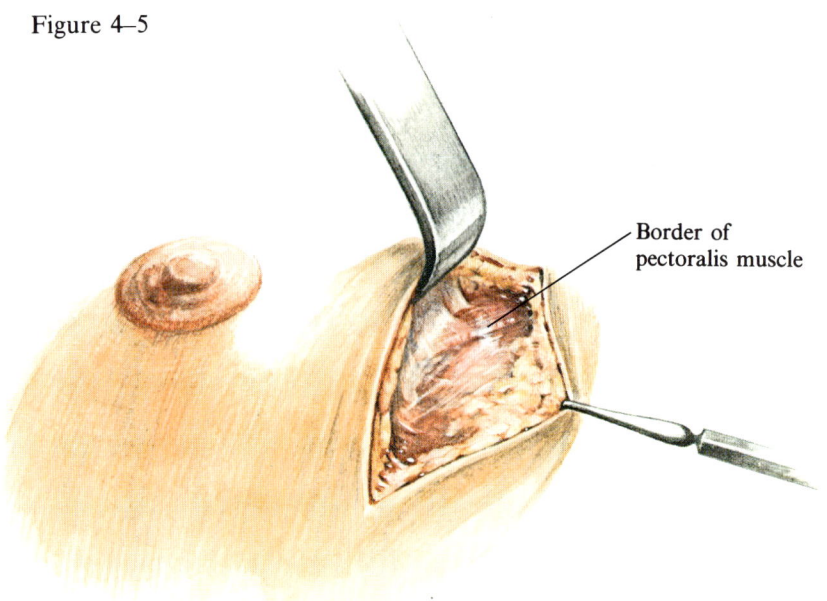

Border of pectoralis muscle

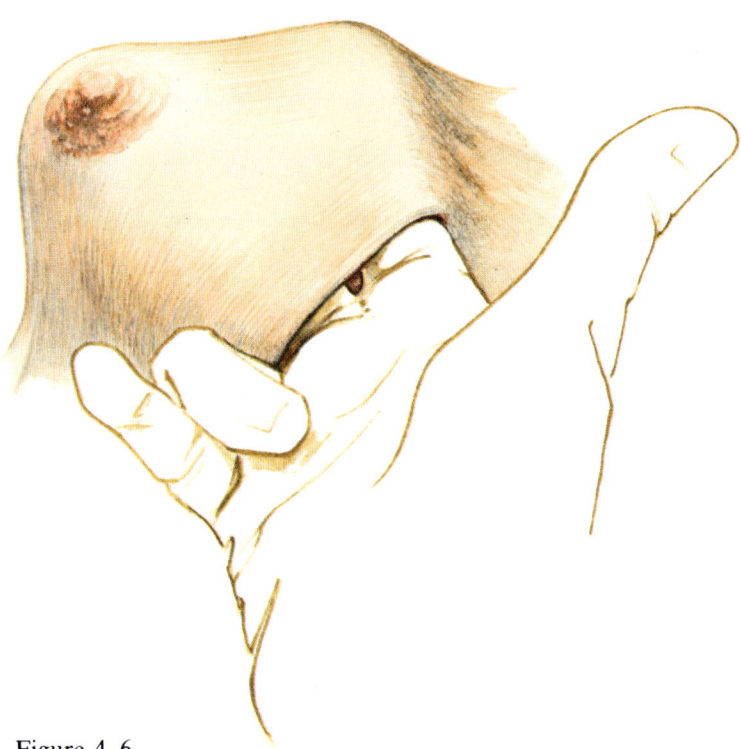

Figure 4–6

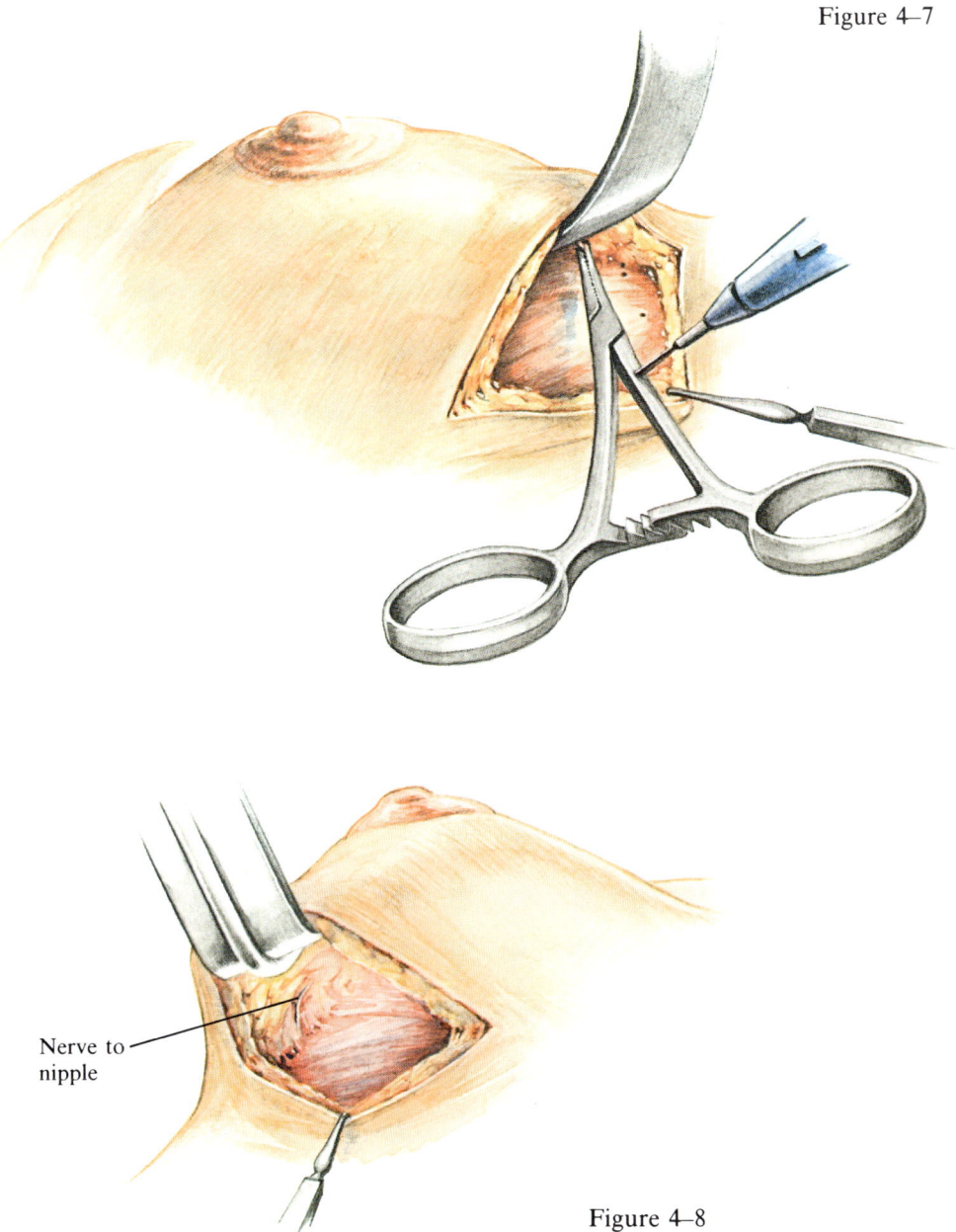

Figure 4–7

Figure 4–8

5. Always dissect the medial and lateral extent of the pocket under direct visualization. Perforating branches of the internal mammary artery must be seen and coagulated prior to division (Fig. 4–7). Retracted vessels are difficult to clamp. The nerve to the nipple passes through the lateral fibrous bands between the serratus anterior muscle and the lateral border of the breast (Fig. 4–8). As the pocket dissection is completed, bleeding ought to be minimal if vessels have been anticipated and coagulated. You may now pause, insert a laparotomy pad, and go on to dissect the other side.
6. Completion follows irrigation with saline, and prolonged examination of the pocket for bleeders. Accumulation of blood along the lateral gutter is indication that a vessel is active somewhere. Also look for loosened fat globules during irrigation. They are devascularized and must be removed so they will not serve as a locus for bacterial proliferation. Avoid infection; leave no ischemic tissue behind.

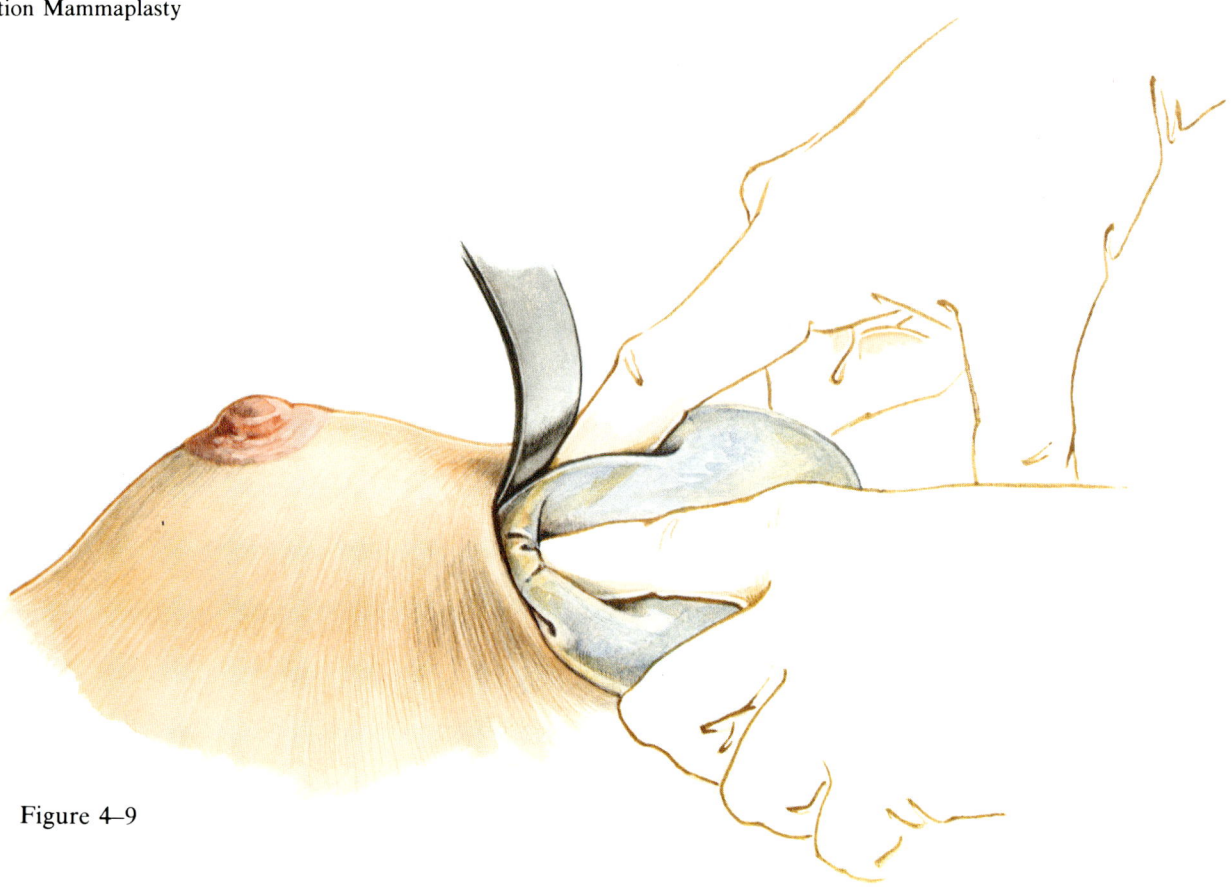

Figure 4-9

7. Now insert the implant (Fig. 4-9). Use a presterilized "sizer" implant if you wish, or if you are certain of the size, proceed to insert the actual transplant. Leave a smooth-bladed retractor in the wound and moisten the implant. Insertion becomes easier with practice. If the implant does not move around in the pocket easily, if it bulges from the incision, or if you can visually delineate the borders of the pocket externally, then either the implant must be replaced with a smaller one or the pocket must be made larger (Fig. 4-10).

8. Prior to closure, insert a single finger, retract the implant medially, and take a final look at the lateral gutter. There must be no accumulation of blood! If there is, remove the implant and repeat the hemostasis routine. Close the incision with buried absorbable sutures, as elsewhere *avoiding injury to the implant.* Approximate skin with a running buried pullout 4-0 prolene suture (Fig. 4-11). Apply a bulky gauze and circumferential Ace bandage dressing, or if you prefer, ask your patient to apply her own bra; line it with gauze pads.

9. Postoperative care includes the following: Bulky dressings are unnecessary after a day. Check for hematomas and nipple sensitivity on the day following surgery. Change dressing daily. Reapply bra immediately with gauze pads. Advise patient to limit activity 2-4 weeks (no lifting, reaching, strenuous sports). Breast massage begins 14 days after surgery. This is based on the rationale that breast softness depends on maintaining the dimensions of the dissected pocket. Patients are asked to use the flat of their hand and press the augmented breast, first superiorly, then medially, then laterally. Many surgeons advise massage for 1 year. Some recommend oral vitamin E in hopes that its glucocorticoid-like effect will reduce the tendency to capsule contraction. No conclusive evidence exists for the effectiveness of either massage or vitamin E. Many patients develop capsule contraction despite all precautions to the contrary.

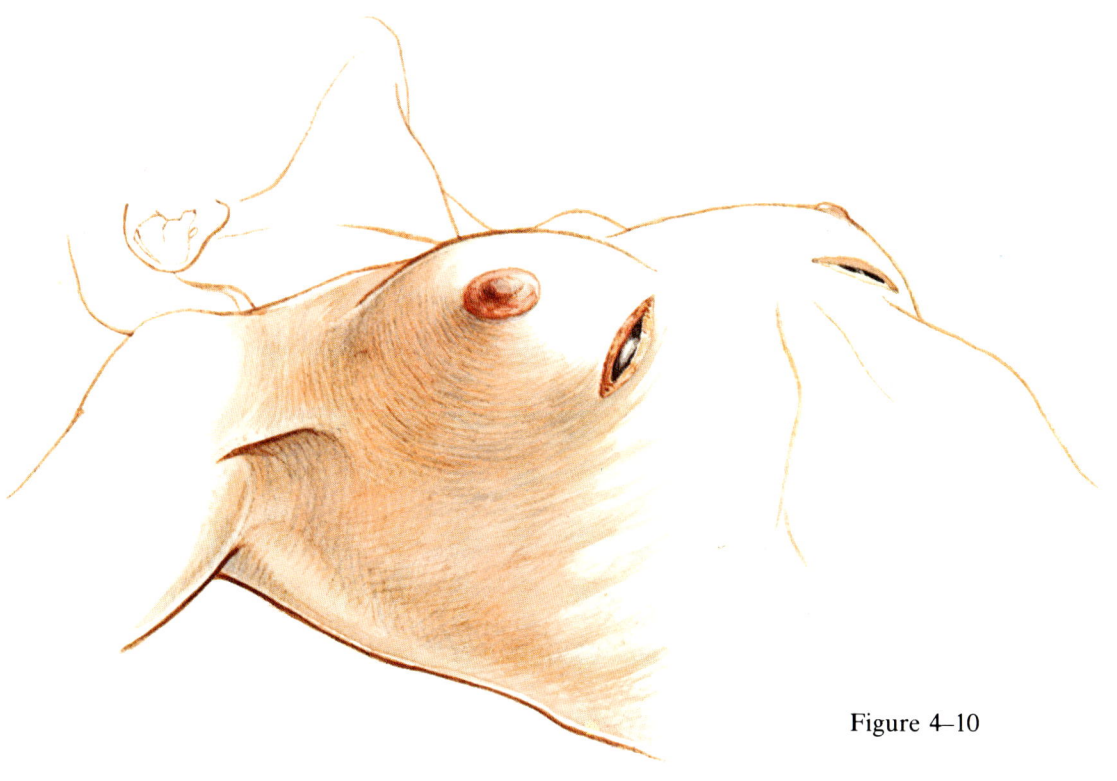

Figure 4–10

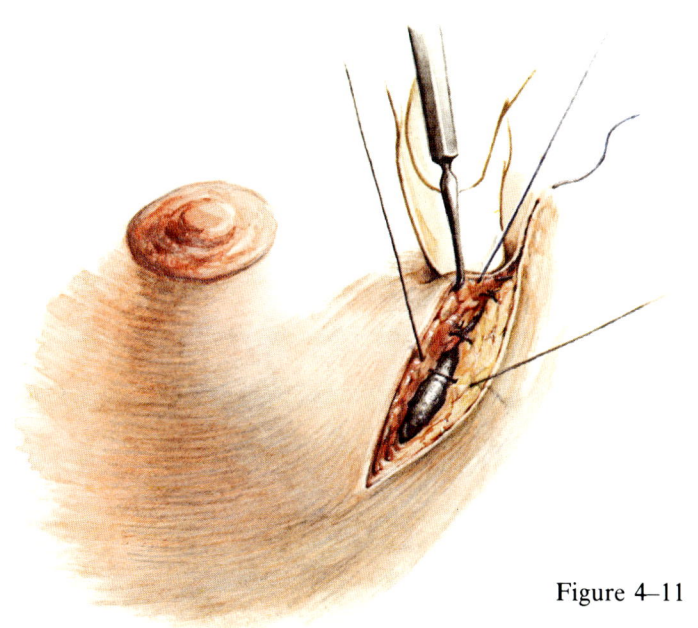

Figure 4–11

Variations

Implant Style

Early implants were designed to simulate normal breast contour. Surgeons and manufacturers later realized that the shape of a female breast is determined by the overlying skin, not the content of the breast. The type of implant used depends on surgeon preference, but most select a round, low-profile, soft-gel, or a double-lumen implant that assumes a breast contour when patients sit or stand.

Initially, silicone implants were solid gel. Subsequently, saline, inflatable, and double-lumen (gel surrounded by a saline-inflatable compartment) implants became popular. Probably the most critical decision regarding implant selection is size. Other variables are less important in determining results.

Periareolar Incision

Whenever the patient is concerned about visibility of the inframammary scar, the periareolar incision is an acceptable alternative. The lower one-half of the areola is used. A circumferential incision is made just inside the perimeter (Fig. 4–12A). Loss of nipple sensation may occur but in practice this is rare. Interruption of milk ducts is also possible, but can be avoided. The healed areolar scar is quite favorable, but still visible.

After incision of areolar and subcutaneous tissue, the dissection is carried through the breast, or if lactation is desired in the future, around the the lower edge of the gland (Fig. 4–12B). After the pectoralis fascia is reached, the pocket is digitally dissected. A fiberoptic retractor is essential for visualizing the limits of dissection, and for achieving hemostasis. Care must be taken to identify the appropriate inferior limit of dissection in the absence of an inframammary incision.

Subpectoral Implantation

Placement of the implant beneath the pectoralis major muscle has been advocated for reducing the frequency of hardened breasts (Fig. 4–13). This is

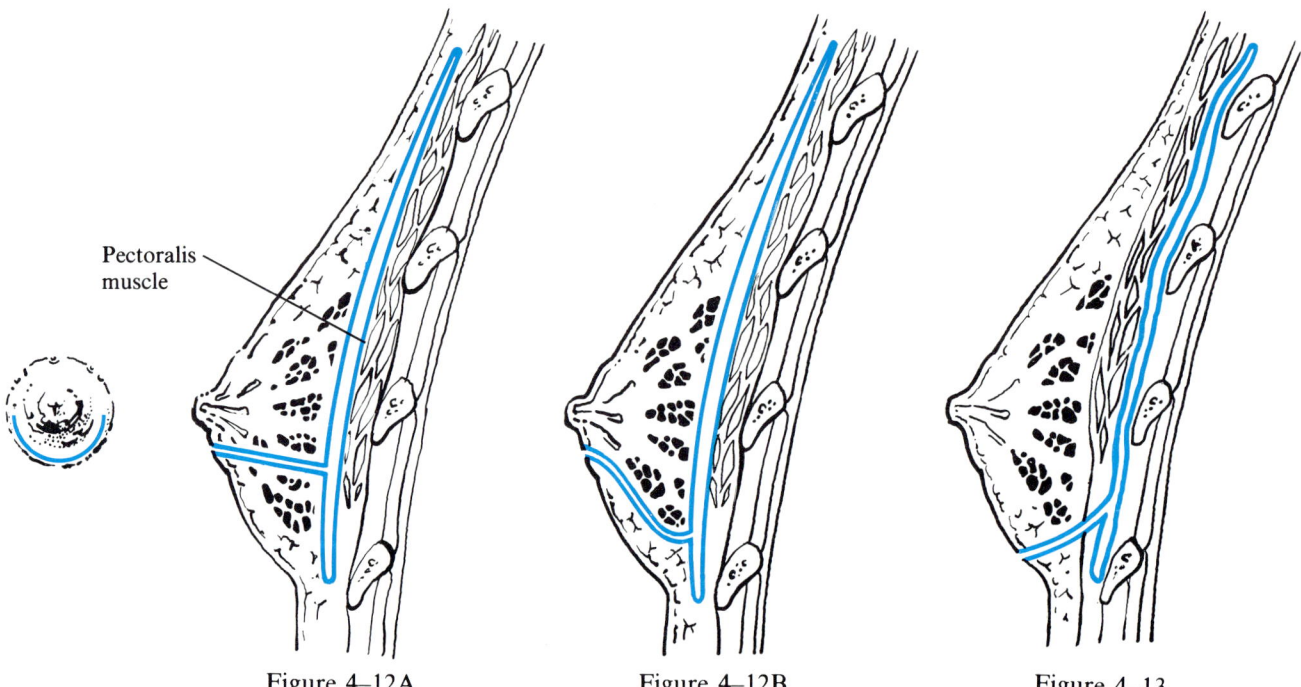

Figure 4–12A   Figure 4–12B   Figure 4–13

still controversial (see Issues), but some insist that the constant action of the muscle maintains the pocket and keeps the breast softer. Others dislike the linear breast distortion that occurs with pectoralis contraction. Other indications for subpectoral implantation include postpartum atrophy and a desire for more fullness above the nipple line. Subpectoral augmentation is usually completed through an inframammary incision. It is easier to slip under the free edge of the pectoralis during dissection than it is to stay above the muscle. The subpectoral plane is essentially bloodless and a generous space can be developed. Using electrocautery, the sternal and costal origins of the pectoralis major are divided to the fourth intercostal space. Perforating branches of the internal mammary artery must be identified and ligated during this portion of the dissection. Do not join the two pockets in midline. Laterally, avoid injury to the nerve supplying the nipple.

Issues

The principal controversy associated with breast augmentation is whether breast firmness can be prevented. This problem is confounding because hardness may develop early or several years following surgery, unilaterally or bilaterally, and following use of gel or saline inflatable implants. The common mechanism in each and every case of breast firmness is implant compression following capsule contraction, the latter presumably mediated by presence of contractile myofibroblasts.

Few if any surgeons still use dacron-backed implants, and use of steroids within the inflatable implant is unpopular. Softer gels may have been associated with more frequent capsule contraction, leading to the hypothesis that silicone "bleed" leads to firmness. However, low-bleed implants do not appear to be the effective answer. Subclinical infection was a popular hypothesis, leading to the use of intraluminal, intrawound antibiotics (or antibiotic foam). Subpectoral implantation is currently popular.

The safest conclusion is that no technique yet proposed has been shown to reliably prevent capsule contraction. Nor does anyone understand why the process occurs. Until we learn more, we must presume that capsule contraction is a variant of normal healing. All patients must therefore be advised to expect some breast firmness following breast augmentation if they wish to avoid disappointment following surgery.

Additional Reading

Lalardrie JP and Mouly R. History of mammaplasty. Aesth Plast Surg 2:167–176, 1978.

Cholonky T. Augmentation mammaplasty. Plast Reconstr Surg 45:573–577, 1970. (A survey of complications observed in 10,941 patients.)

Biggs TM, Cukier J, Worthing LF. Augmentation mammaplasty: A review of 18 years. Plast Reconstr Surg 69:445–452, 1982. (A more recent analysis of experience with 1567 patients by one surgical group.)

Rudolph R, Abraham J, Vecchione T, Guber S, and Woodward M. Myofibroblasts and free silicon around breast implants. Plast Reconstr Surg 62:185–196, 1978. (Both contractile myofibroblasts and free silicon particles can be found in breast implant capsules.)

Breast Reduction/ Elevation

5

Carson M. Lewis and Jack C. Fisher

Background

The problem of oversized breasts was first approached surgically by Gaillard-Thomas in 1882. He removed a disc of glandular tissue from the base of the breast. Morestin and De Quervain improved on the technique, but nipple ptosis remained an unsolved problem.

Thorek in 1922 and Lexer in 1925 combined glandular reduction with free transplantation of the nipple. This technique remains in use today.

The modern era of breast reduction began with Beisenberger, who, in 1928, offered a method for reshaping the breast that remained after glandular reduction. His technique required considerable undermining of skin, a significant disadvantage. Schwartzman in 1936 described a safe means for preserving nipple viability during glandular reduction. Many others refined Biesenberger's method during and after World War II. Not until 1957 did Aries demonstrate how a breast could be reduced and the nipple elevated without endangering viability of the nipple or the breast skin. Since that time, the refinements of Wiener, and of McKissock have provided a more precise definition of and method for reliably preserving nerve and blood supply of the nipple.

Today, the principles for reducing the oversized breast and elevating the ptotic breast are basically the same. The only essential difference is excision of glandular tissue. These procedures are discussed together in Chapter 2.

Indications

Medical

1. Discomfort due to oversized breasts, e.g., pain, postural change, skin rash (Fig. 5–1)

Aesthetic

2. Embarrassment and deformity due to oversized breasts
3. Ptosis, secondary to hypertrophy, pregnancy, or obesity.

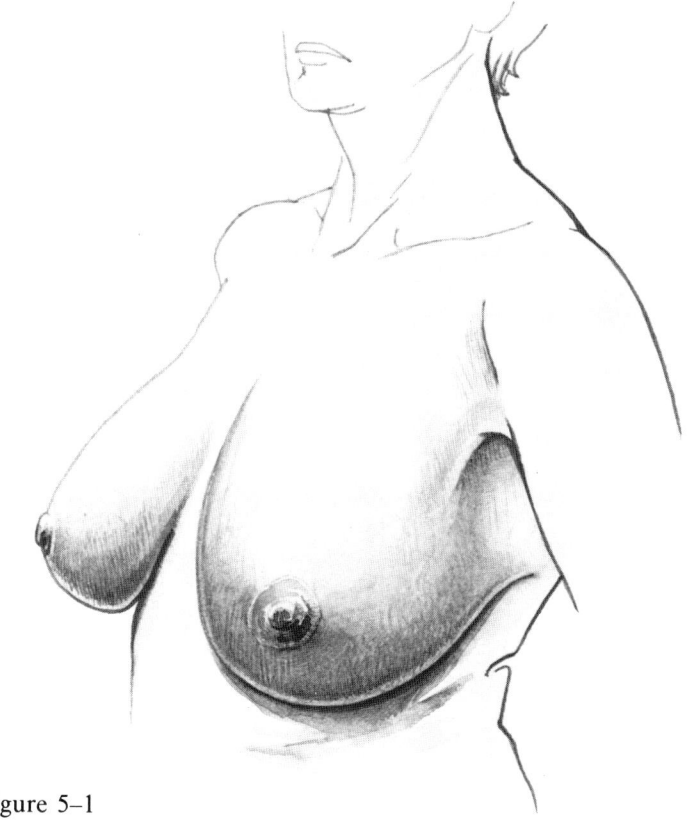

Figure 5–1

Contraindications

Absolute

1. Unwillingness to accept scars or possible loss of nipple sensitivity
2. Unrealistic expectations

Relative

1. Untreated obesity (begin weight reduction program before surgery)
2. Silicone mastitis
3. Clinical signs of breast malignancy (biopsy first)
4. High risk of cancer (consider subcutaneous mastectomy).

What the Patient Needs to Know Before Surgery

Will Occur

1. Scars: Indicate their location (breast scars are always wider than facial scars). The require 6–12 months for maturation and may require injection or revision.

Can Occur

1. Asymmetry of breast size, shape, or nipple position
2. Nipple ischemia
3. Nipple anesthesia

4. Nipples may not project
5. Skin loss at corners of skin flaps (5 to 10%)
6. Fat necrosis, delayed healing, infection (2–5%).

What the Surgeon Must Know

Breast Topography

Surgeons must be familiar with the shape of the skin of the normal (and pendulous) breast. Remember that the shape of the female breast is determined by the overlying skin, not by the underlying gland. The plastic surgeon determines the shape of the patient's breast by preoperative design and intraoperative flap manipulation.

Nipple position in the *young* woman with normal breasts is 17–19 cm from the sternal notch. But for women with breast enlargement or ptosis, inferior displacement of the breasts exists, not all of which can or should be corrected. Therefore, select a nipple position 20–22 cm from the sternal notch for best results.

Nipple Blood Supply

Understand well the several sources of blood supply to the nipple. These include (a) the posterior intercostal arteries, (b) the perforating branches of the internal mammary artery, and (c) the lateral thoracic branch of the axillary artery. By the time blood reaches the nipple, it courses through branches within the breast itself, in the overlying subcutaneous layers, and in the subdermal plexus of the skin. Do not, therefore, engage in arguments about the importance of preserving dermis adjacent to the nipple. The dermis most certainly is contributory, but not exclusively so. Either a superior or an inferior pedicle can reliably support a nipple, particularly when the nipple retains some attachment to the underlying breast. If this is not possible, two pedicles are probably better than one. In other words, your goal is to preserve sufficient blood supply. Pedicle length is not a reliable index for success; the manner of dissection and the thickness of the pedicle are also important. These are matters of technical judgement to be learned from wise supervision and experience, not from books or numerical rules.

Nipple Nerve Supply

Know the innervation of the nipple. These are the anterior and lateral perforating branches of the third, fourth, and fifth intercostal nerves, and the supraclavicular branch of the cervical plexus. Do all you can to preserve nipple sensitivity. The breast is a nourishing organ only during childbearing years. It is an organ of sexuality for the remainder of your patient's life. She will not relinquish nipple sensitivity willingly unless required to do so for the severest deformities.

Screening for Breast Disease

Finally, be aware of community standards for determining the presence of primary breast disease. Be thorough in your physical examination of the breast. Work closely with a surgical oncologist who knows how to manage mastodynia and fibrocystic disease, or how to biopsy and manage breast carcinoma. In return, you obtain referrals for postmastectomy reconstruction, and the patient receives valuable reassurance before an elective breast procedure. Do not forget a mammogram following breast reduction (recommended by breast cancer surgeons as a baseline examination for comparison with future mammograms).

Breast Reduction/Elevation

Operative Design

More than for any other operation described in this book, the success of breast reduction is a derivative of careful design and preoperative marking.

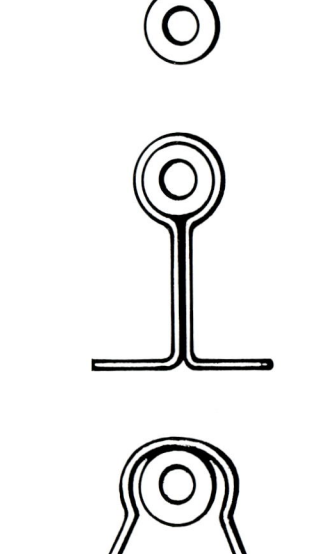

Figure 5–2A

1. *Always* mark a patient while she is sitting upright. Use a warm, quiet, and private place. Take your time. The patient will become more reassured and confident as she observes the care with which you measure and mark her breasts. A rush job will not be overlooked by the patient.
2. Do not wait until the patient is in the operating room to mark incisions. It is a drafty, busy place, not very private, distractive, and embarrassing for the patient. In this setting, she may overlook your efforts while she deals with her anger and apprehension.
3. Ask your patient not to shower after breast markings are made. Also ask her to reject prep technicians and nurses who might seem compelled to wash off markings based on habits learned on other surgical services.
4. Marking Sequence:
   a. Suprasternal notch
   b. Midclavicular points
   c. Line from midclavicular to ipsilateral nipple, then down to the midinframammary crease
   d. Line along entire inframammary crease
   e. Select and mark new nipple site
      Guidelines are at the level of the inframammary crease or 19–22 cm from the suprasternal notch (it is better to be too low than too high). Facilitate nipple site marking with appropriate sized washer or with inverted medicine glass; or lay the flexible wire pattern (Fig. 5–2A) that makes flap design easier.

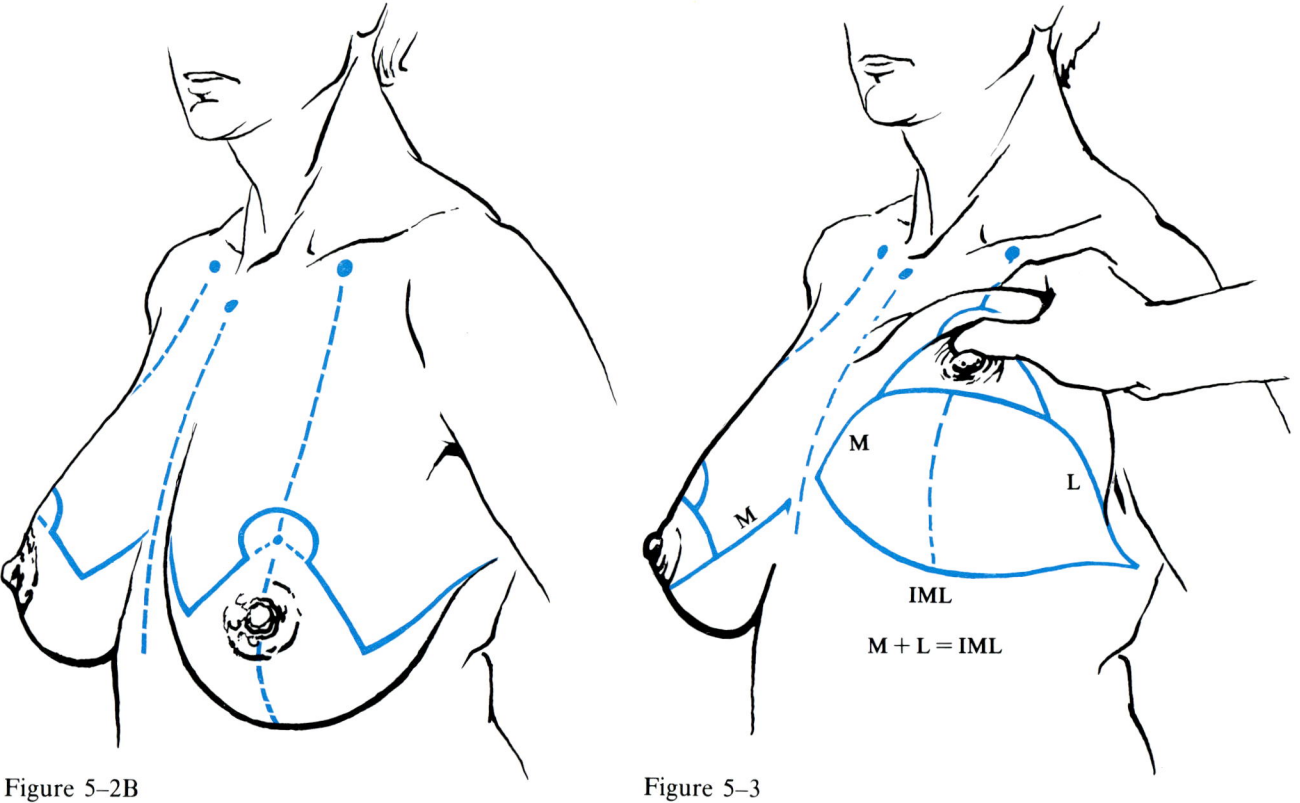

Figure 5–2B

Figure 5–3

f. Duplicate all marks on the other side. Never connect two inframammary incisions in the midline; a scar web will result.
   g. Now draw the areolar margin around each new nipple site.
   h. Outline breast flaps. Extend a vertical incision inferiorly from nipple, either side of areola; vertical height of flap should be no less than 5 cm, no more than 6 cm (Fig. 5–2B).
   i. Now join vertical margin with inframammary line. Some prefer a sigmoid line to extend flap length, and avoid dogears. Length of medial flap (M) and length of lateral flap (L) must equal length of inframammary line (IML) (Fig. 5–3).
   j. Step back, check carefully, confirm all measurements and markings; nipple sites have to be at the same level.
5. After patient is anesthetized, scratch center of nipple site and midpoint of the inframammary crease as a permanent mark. Reinforce nipple and flap markings with marking solution (Fig. 5–4).
6. Ask the nurse to prep the skin gently, but not to erase marks.
7. Drape.
8. Begin infiltration of skin with epinephrine diluted 1:200,000. If necessary, reinforce nipple and flap marks once again before beginning.

Anesthesia

1. Most reduction mammoplasties require general anesthesia.
2. There is patient benefit and cost advantage to having assistance; a double team permits simultaneous breast correction and limits anesthesia time.
3. Avoid blood loss and transfusion. Use diluted epinephrine (1:200,000) to control dermal bleeding. Request electrocautery for each operating team. When breasts are enormous, anticipate blood loss and schedule autotransfusion in advance.
4. Breast elevation (mastopexy) without gland excision can be done safely under local block when the patient is adequately prepared and sedated.

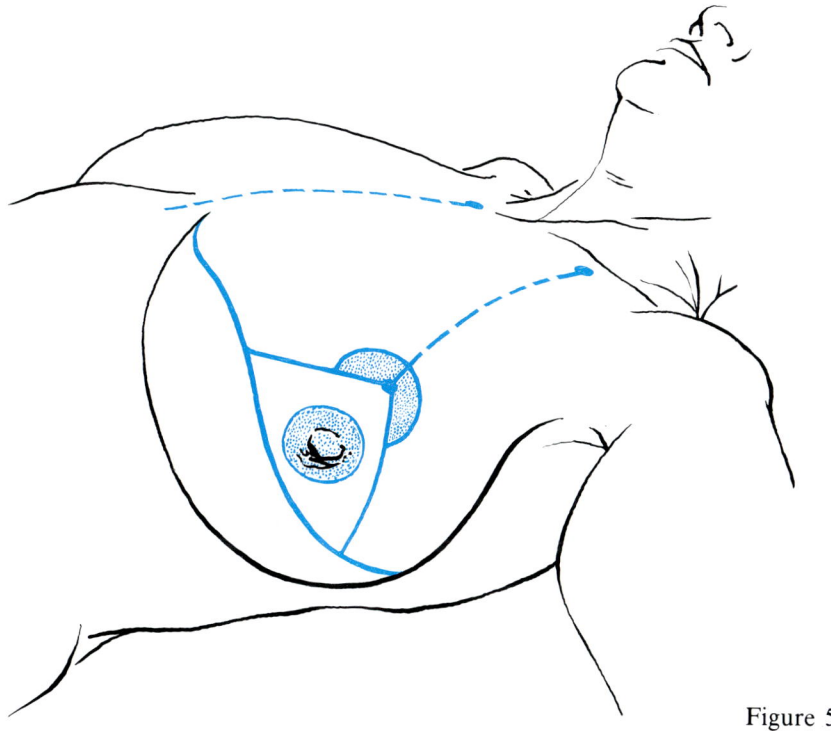

Figure 5–4

Operative Technique

Described below is the classic and still useful method: reduction with free nipple grafts. Afterward the variations can be learned and perfected. This procedure is applicable to the very large-breasted woman, or the patient for whom preservation of nipple sensitivity is not important. You will enjoy the greatest intraoperative flexibility with this procedure. Nipple viability is ensured if you graft accurately. No pedicles need be preserved or manipulated.

1. Recheck and reinforce marks. Communicate your plan to the contralateral team. Whatever is done, do it the same on both sides. Always remember that symmetry is important!
2. Remove nipple-areola complex quickly as free graft, including dermis and fat (Fig. 5–5); store tissue on back table wrapped in saline-soaked gauze.
3. Incise all premarked flap margins.
4. Excise full thickness skin and subcutaneous tissue from inside the premarked breast flap margins (Fig. 5–6).
5. Achieve hemostasis; then dissect the breast from the pectoralis fascia up to a level well above the new nipple site (Fig. 5–7).

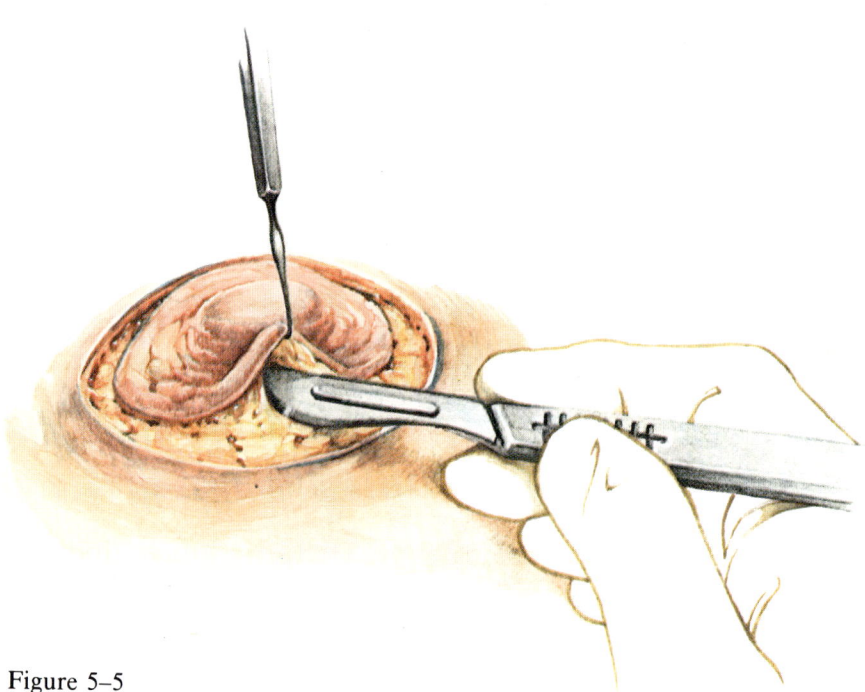

Figure 5–5

Operative Technique

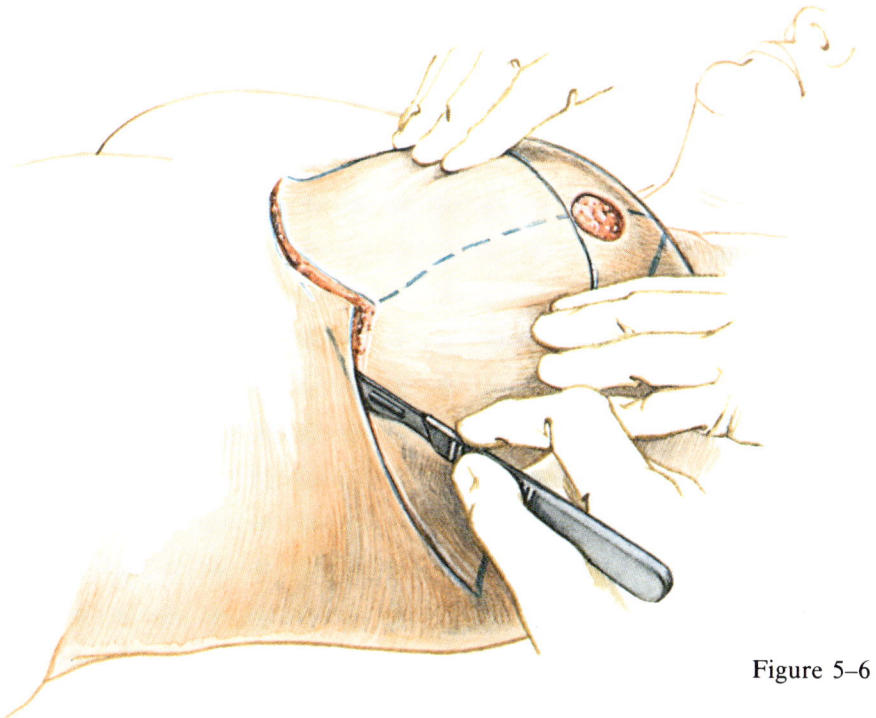

Figure 5–6

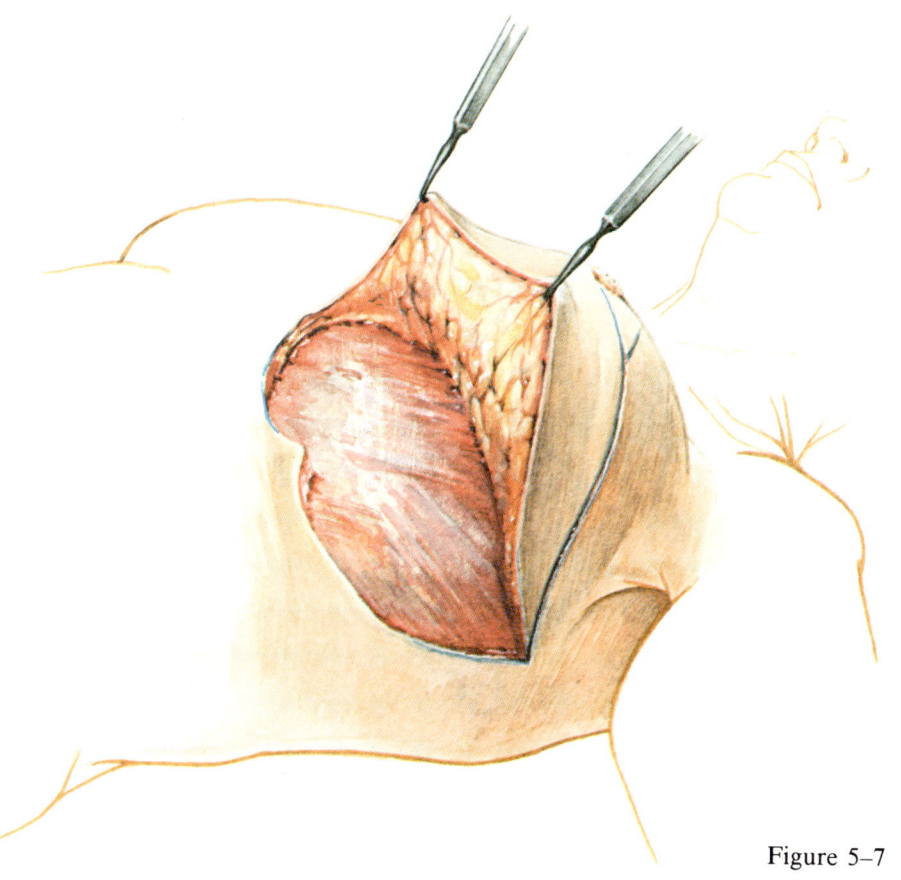

Figure 5–7

31

Breast Reduction/Elevation

6. Excise wedge of breast tissue from the inferior quadrant in a quantity sufficient to satisfy the patient's goal (Fig. 5–8). Extend the wedge superior to the new nipple site (Fig. 5–9). Then thin medial and lateral flaps. Be conservative with the medial flap, liberal with the lateral flap (Fig. 5–10).

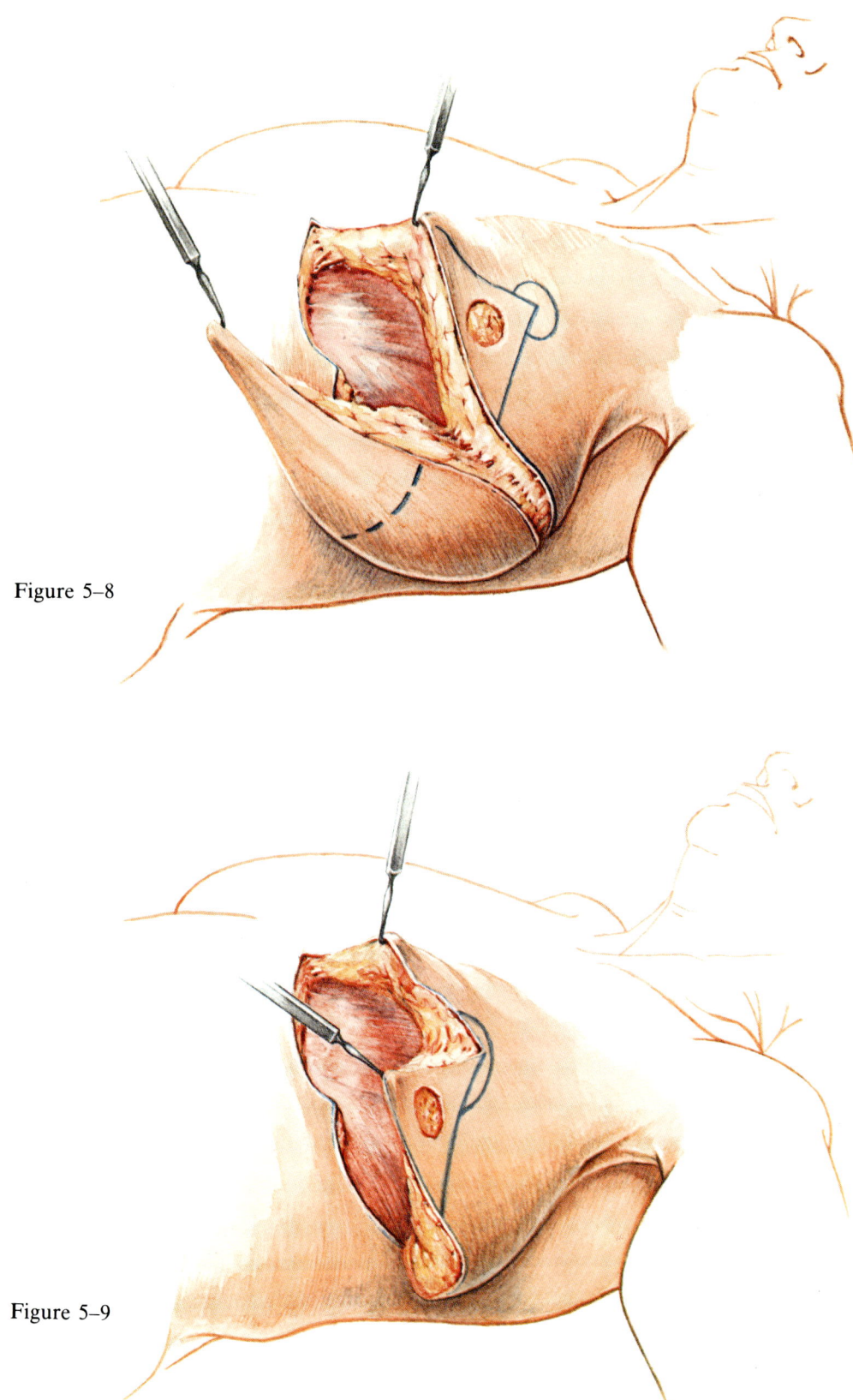

Figure 5–8

Figure 5–9

7. Remind the scrub nurse to keep right and left specimens separate for independent weighing. Also transmit specimens to the pathologist individually.
8. Achieve hemostasis. Irrigate wounds.
9. Place trial suture (3–0 absorbable) to approximate medial and lateral flaps to premarked midpoint of the inframammary margin (Fig. 5–11).

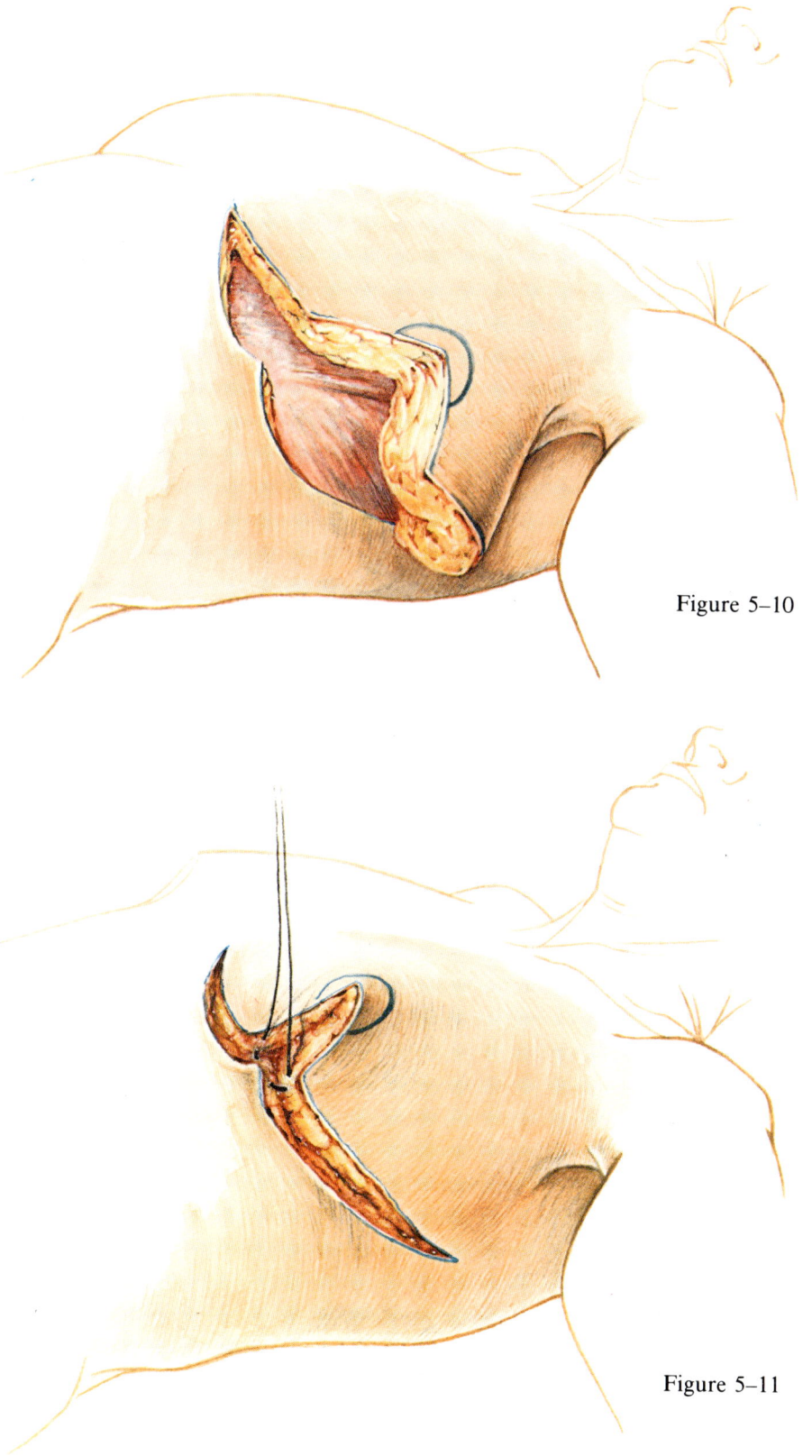

Figure 5–10

Figure 5–11

10. Reevaluate breast site and shape. Make revisions; excise tissue to achieve symmetry. Compare weights of excised tissue as an additional guide.
11. Approximate medial and lateral breast flaps in midline and along the inframammary crease. Close from lateral to medial to minimize lateral "dog ears." Shorten flaps medially as needed to achieve a conical breast.
12. Remove only the epithelium from new nipple site, leaving a dermal bed for the nipple areola graft (Figs. 5–12 and 5–13).
13. Now defat the graft, excising fat and some dermis (Fig. 5–14). Preserve some breast tissue beneath the nipple to assure nipple projection.
14. Suture nipple/areola graft to dermal bed, and secure with a tie-over dressing (Figs. 5–15, 5–16, 5–17).
15. Close the skin incisions with a running subcuticular pullout suture (to minimize cross-hatching); reinforce with adhesive strips.
16. Drains may be used if desired. Bring them out at the lateral end of the inframammary wound, not a separate drain site. This avoids unnecessary extra scars!

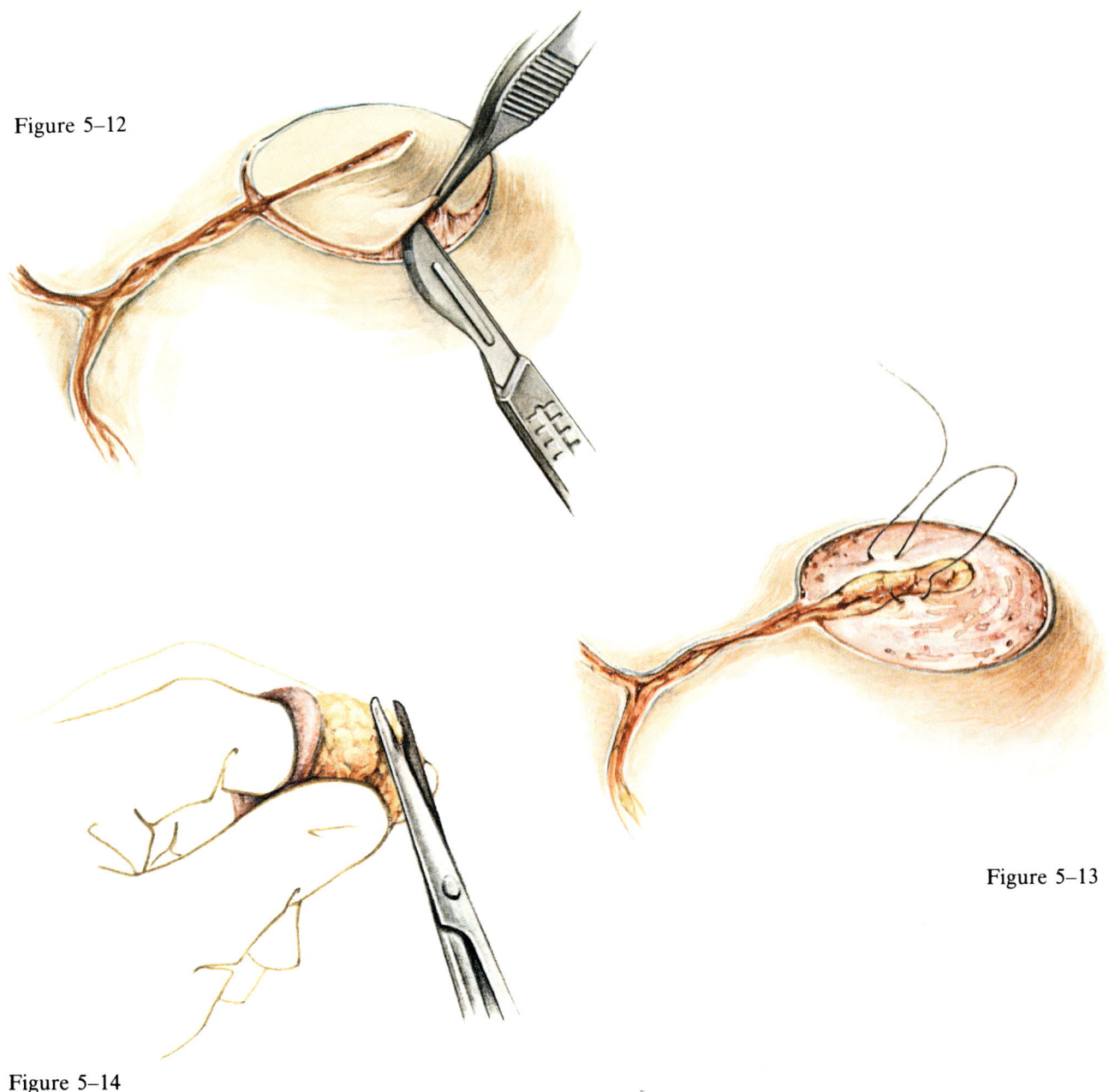

Figure 5–12

Figure 5–13

Figure 5–14

Operative Technique

Figure 5–15

Figure 5–16

Figure 5–17

35

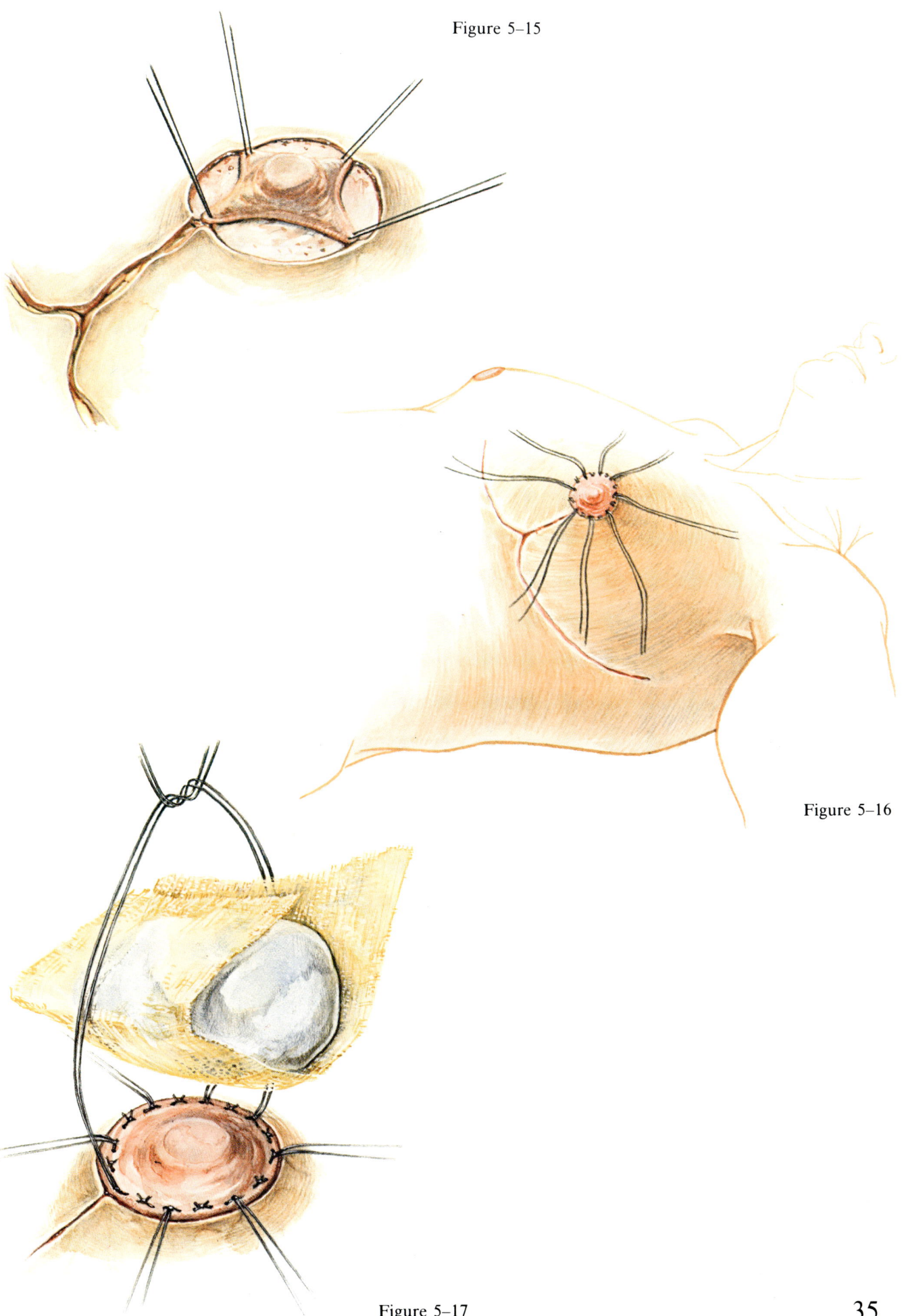

Variations

You have been shown a basic procedure that incorporates redesign of the breast skin envelope with the ability to remove any amount of glandular tissue. Other breast reduction procedures are variations on the same theme. Simple breast elevation (mastopexy) is based on similar principles, but without glandular resection and always with preservation of nipple sensation and viability. Below is a list of variations together with pertinent references for further study.

Defining Nipple Placement

A good plastic surgical principle is to defer commitment of tissue until the last possible moment. The basic technique described includes designation of the nipple site at the beginning. A nipple site must be selected and marked initially since all other marks emanate from this point. But the nipple-areola graft can be shifted a few millimeters at the end in order to ensure proper positioning. Often the best result is achieved when the nipple is centered slightly below the conical point of the reduced breast. Avoid placing the nipple too high or you produce the unsightly, and not uncommon, "star gazing nipple."

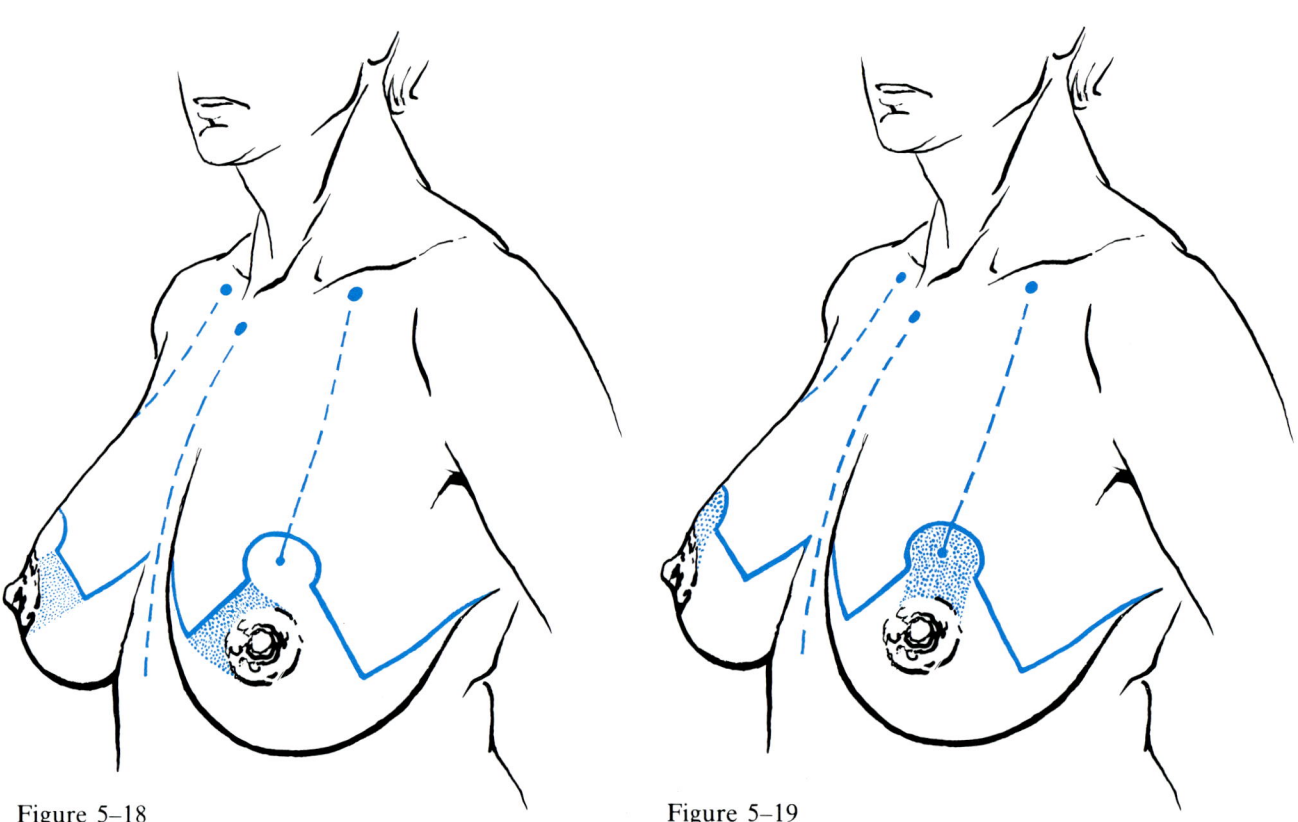

Figure 5–18   Figure 5–19

Variations of Nipple Pedicle
During breast reduction or elevation, the nipple can be safely moved on a variety of pedicles, the essential goal being preservation of both blood and nerve supply. Already discussed are the multiple sources of blood supply to the nipple/areola complex. As might be expected, the literature is filled with variations on breast reduction/elevation based on several acceptable pedicles. Your obligation is to preserve enough blood supply, not to defend the adequacy of one pedicle over another. Therefore, read carefully the following pedicle advocates:

Lateral (or medial) pedicle (Skoog) (Fig. 5–18)
Superior pedicle only (Wiener) (Fig. 5–19)
Vertical bipedicle (McKissock) (Fig. 5–20A and B)
Horizontal bipedicle (Strombeck)
Inferior pedicle only (Robbins)

The advantages and disadvantages of each deserve close scrutiny.

Variations in Flap Design
Other techniques are used for the skin envelope of the corrected breast. These include the methods of Aries/Pitanquy and of Dufourmentel/Schatten.

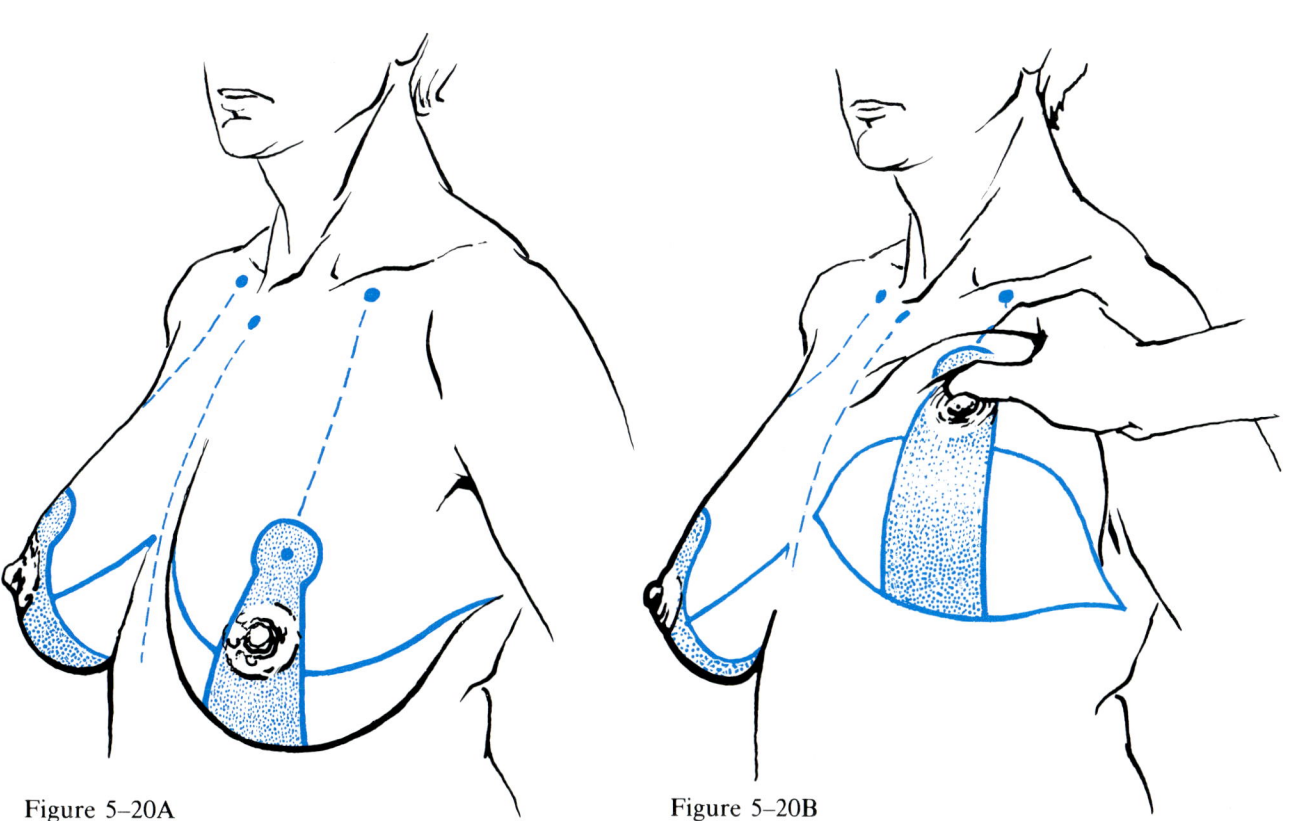

Figure 5–20A Figure 5–20B

Issues

Few, if any, genuine issues exist for breast reduction/elevation. The abundance of literature on this subject is a derivative of multiple variations, sometimes presented as if they represented issues for debate or conquest.

Additional Reading

Lalardrie JP and Mouly R. History of mammaplasty. Aesth Plast Surg 2:167–176, 1978. (Includes a reference list for nearly all the principles and variations of breast reduction and elevation.)

Ramirez M. Normal size and shape of the breast and elaboration of a natural pattern. Aesth Plast Surg 2:383–393, 1978. (A review of available data for preoperative design of a breast reduction or mastopexy.)

Courtiss EH and Goldwyn RM. Breast sensation before and after plastic surgery. Plast Reconstr Surg 58:1–13, 1975. (Anatomic basis for and clinical experience with nipple transposition without loss of function.)

McKissock P. Reduction mammaplasty with a vertical dermal flap. Plast Reconstr Surg 49:245–252, 1972. (Original description of the highly popular vertical bipedicle technique for nipple transposition.)

Weiner DL, Dolich BH, Miclat MI. Reduction mammoplasty utilizing the superior pedicle technique: A six year retrospective. Aesth Plast Surg 6:7–14, 1982.

Wise RJ. A preliminary report on a method of planning the mammaplasty. Plast Reconstr Surg 17:367, 1956.

Strombeck JO. Mammaplasty: Report of a new technique based on the two-pedicle procedure. Brit J Plast Surg 13:79, 1960.

Pitanguy I. Surgical treatment of breast hypertrophy. Brit J Plast Surg 20:78, 1967.

Rees RD. An historical review of reduction mammaplasty, in Hueston JT. (ed): Transactions of the Fifth International Congress of Plastic and Reconstructive Surgery. Butterworth Publications, Sidney, 1971, p 1167.

Schatten WE, Hartley JH, and Hamm WG. Reduction mammaplasty by the Dufourmentel-Mouly method. Plast Reconstr Surg 48:306–310, 1971.

Skoog T. A technique of breast reconstruction: Transposition of the nipple on a cutaneous vascular pedicle. ACTA Chir Scand 126:453, 1963.

Abdominoplasty

Jose Guerrerosantos and Jack C. Fisher

Background

Early descriptions of abdominal wall tightening were offered by general surgeons, willing to trim extra fat and skin. Kelly, Johns Hopkins' eminent gynecologic surgeon, in 1889 resected a large horizontal ellipse of redundant tissue. Rochay removed a trough of tissue from above the umbilicus, and then closed the defect as an inverted "T." Babcock later recommended a vertically oriented resection of skin and fat. Gonzalez-Ulloa expanded the resection principle to the gluteal region. Finally in 1965, Callia demonstrated the advantage of ample abdominal skin undermining and rectus abdominus plication. His procedure is the one we still use today with a few added variations.

Indications

There is one appropriate indication for abdominoplasty, a flaccid abdomen with redundant skin, perhaps also fat accumulation or rectus abdominus diastasis. The deformity, a result of pregnancy and/or obesity, can be categorized according to severity:

1. Mild: lax skin, perhaps stria, some fat accumulation, mild rectus diastasis. This problem can often be treated successfully by diet and exercise.
2. Moderate: redundant skin, rectus diastasis, stria common, significant fat accumulation. These patients need surgery in addition to diet and exercise (Fig. 6–1).
3. Severe: associated with excessive fat deposition. Surgery must be preceded by attention to diet and muscle tone. These patients are often dispirited but their moods can be improved by anticipation of abdomen-tightening surgery.

Potential Contraindications

1. Multiple previous abdominal scars
2. Unwillingness to accept abdominal scars
3. Unrealistic expectations
4. Unstable medical status
5. Psychologic instability.

Abdominoplasty

What the Patient Needs to Know Before Surgery

1. The surgeon improves the shape of the abdomen by removing redundant skin, trimming fat modestly, and tightening underlying muscles. The operation requires 2–3 h for completion.
2. Scars are permanent and lie very low in the abdomen. Patients are encouraged to discuss bathing suit fashions before surgery; they must know where scars will be located. A scar will encircle the umbilicus, and may occasionally extend vertically from umbilicus to suprapubic region.

What the Surgeon Must Know

1. Blood supply to the abdominal wall is abundant, making infection rare but seroma and hematoma more common. Skin of the abdomen is nourished by (a) segmental perforating branches of the subcostal, intercostal,

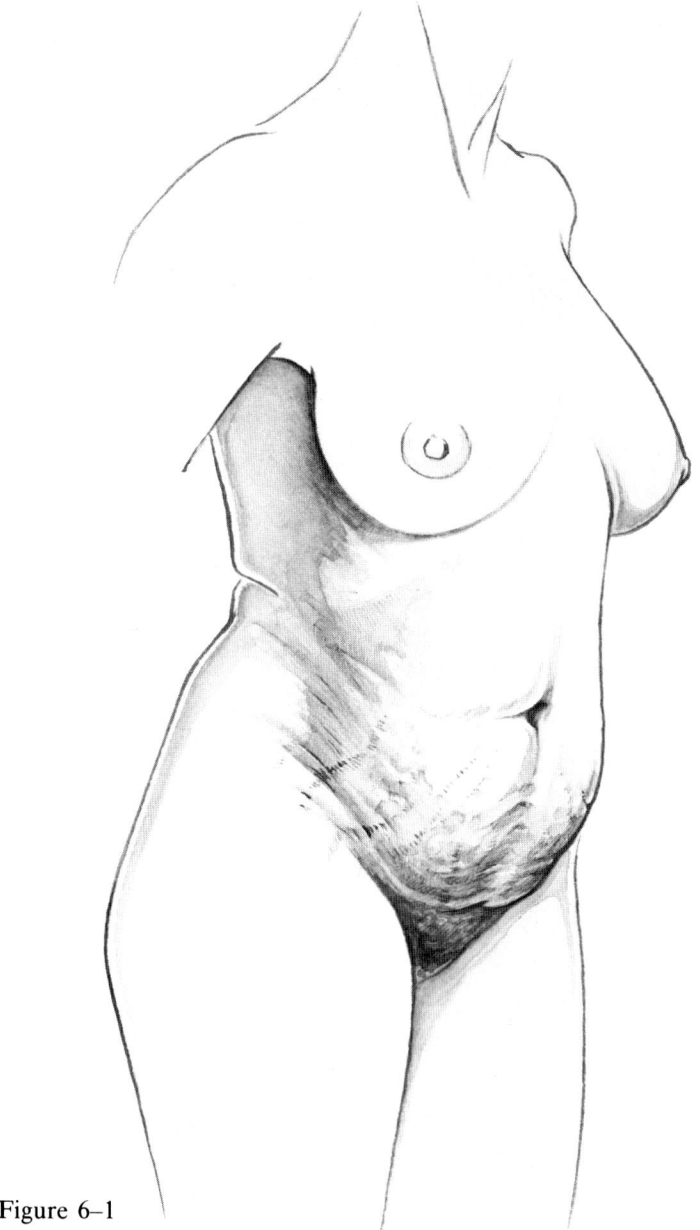

Figure 6–1

and lumbar arteries; (b) superior and inferior epigastric perforators of the rectus abdominus sheath; and (c) superficial branches of the femoral artery. Venous drainage varies somewhat, but generally parallels arterial supply.
2. Cutaneous nerve supply of the abdominal wall includes intercostal nerves, spinal branches of T6 to T12, and the ilioinguinal and ilioliypogastric nerves. Following abdominoplasty, the dermatomes are altered.
3. Patient anatomic variations: examine carefully for umbilical or other herniae, rectus diastasis, prior scars, or skin pathology.
4. Prior incisions above the umbilicus, e.g., for intestinal bypass, may limit vascularity of the abdominal skin flap.
5. Patients are hospitalized 2–5 days following abdominoplasty.
6. Striae cannot be fully removed; only those located in the lower abdomen will be taken with the removed skin segment.
7. Patients will initially feel "bent over" as they walk following surgery; this feeling disappears in 7–14 days.
8. Edema of the abdominal skin and subcutaneous fat will persist for several weeks after surgery, perhaps making patients temporarily disappointed. This swelling will pass with time.
9. Potential complications include fluid accumulation (seroma), hematoma, and delayed healing due to wound separation or skin loss.
10. Less common complications include infection, conspicuous umbilical scar, umbilical stenosis, asymmetry or umbilical position, redundant lower abdomen and skin folds, and cutaneous anesthesia.
11. Pulmonary embolism has been encountered following abdominoplasty but it is uncommon.

Operative Planning

1. Mark abdomen while patient is standing. Estimate skin excision by traction of redundant skin fold. Mark a vertical dotted line from xyphoid process to mid-pubic point.
2. The transverse incision is located in midline 2 cm above the pubis or slightly higher. It follows the inguinal crease laterally and ends short of the anterior superior iliac spine.
3. Mark an oval periumbilical incision.
4. Estimate with a dotted line the undermined zone. This should reach above the costal margin. Also dot in the inferior zone of undermining (see Fig. 6–2).
5. Patients with a more severe deformity may benefit from a higher resection and therefore higher incision. In other words, remove the most redundant tissue with the least undermining. Scar placement is less of a concern in postobesity deformity.

Anesthesia

Abdominoplasty is usually done with the assistance of general anesthesia. A high epidural anesthetic can at times be sufficient with supplemental local infiltration at the superior extent of the dissection but this is impractical most of the time. Those patients having corrective surgery after extraordinary weight loss must receive thorough evaluation of liver function prior to administration of general anesthesia.

Abdominoplasty

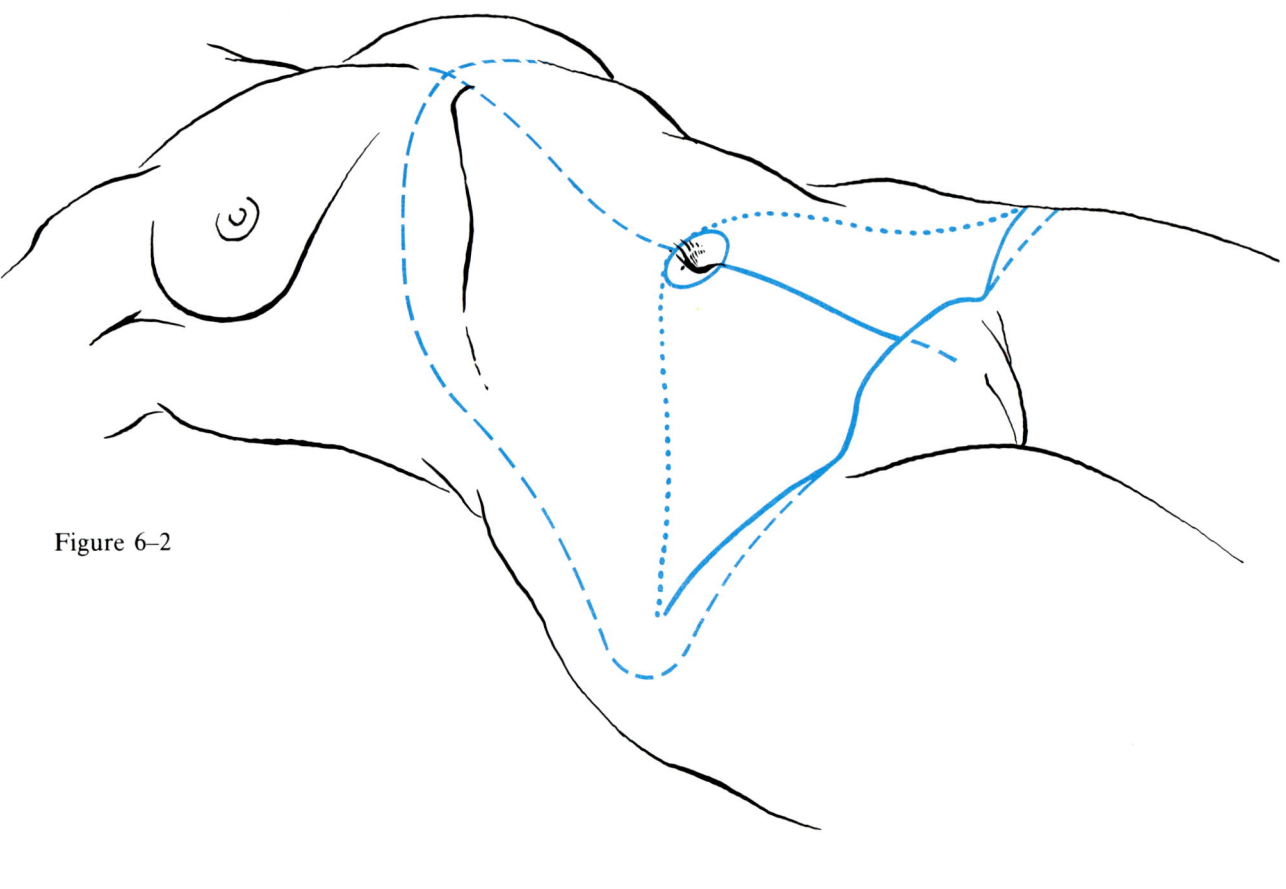

Figure 6–2

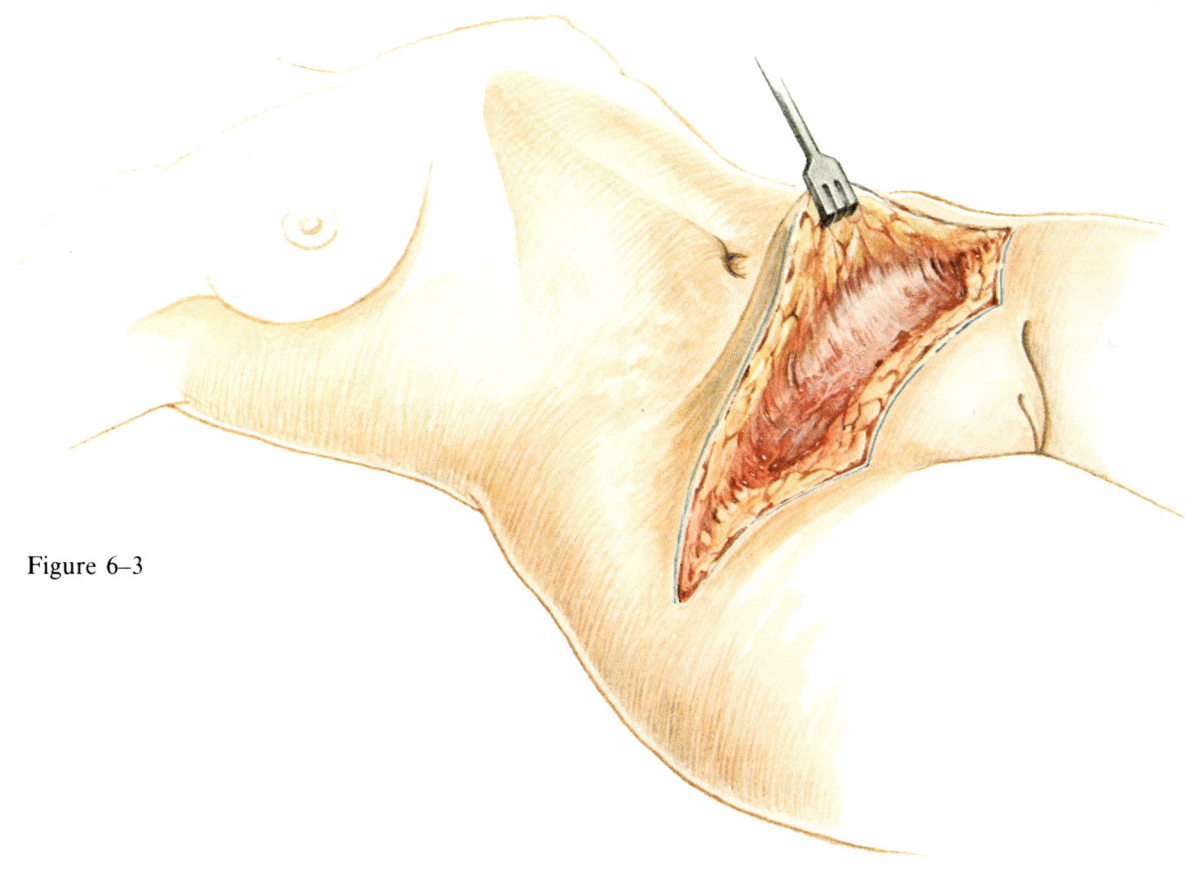

Figure 6–3

42

Operative Technique

1. Flex patient slightly even before you begin. Be certain patient is positioned on table appropriately to permit additional flexing prior to closure.
2. Incise lower abdominal skin. Following hemostatis, extend depth of wound in midline nearly to the fascia. Begin to dissect superiorly, separating abdominal flap from fascia. Remain in the loose areolar layer rather than dissect at the fascia surface (Fig. 6–3). This way, perforating vessels can be spotted more easily, clamped, and coagulated before they retract into fascia.
3. Laterally, undermine skin more superficially, and leave some subcutaneous fat or fascia in order to assist preservation of lymphatics and cutaneous nerve supply.
4. As dissection proceeds superiorly and the umbilicus is approached, pause and make a periumbilical incision (Fig. 6–4). Dissect entire umbilicus free of abdominal skin down to the fascia level. Divide flap in midline, inferior to umbilical site; this facilitates exposure during the remainder of the dissection (Fig. 6–5).

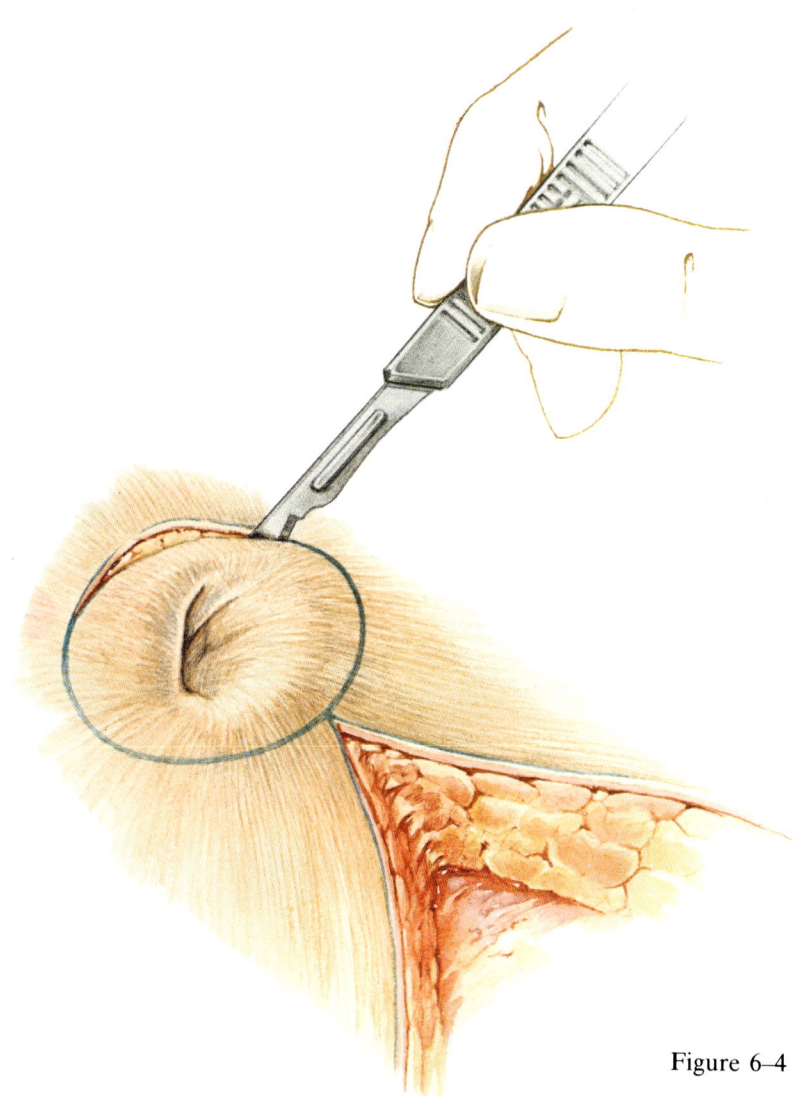

Figure 6–4

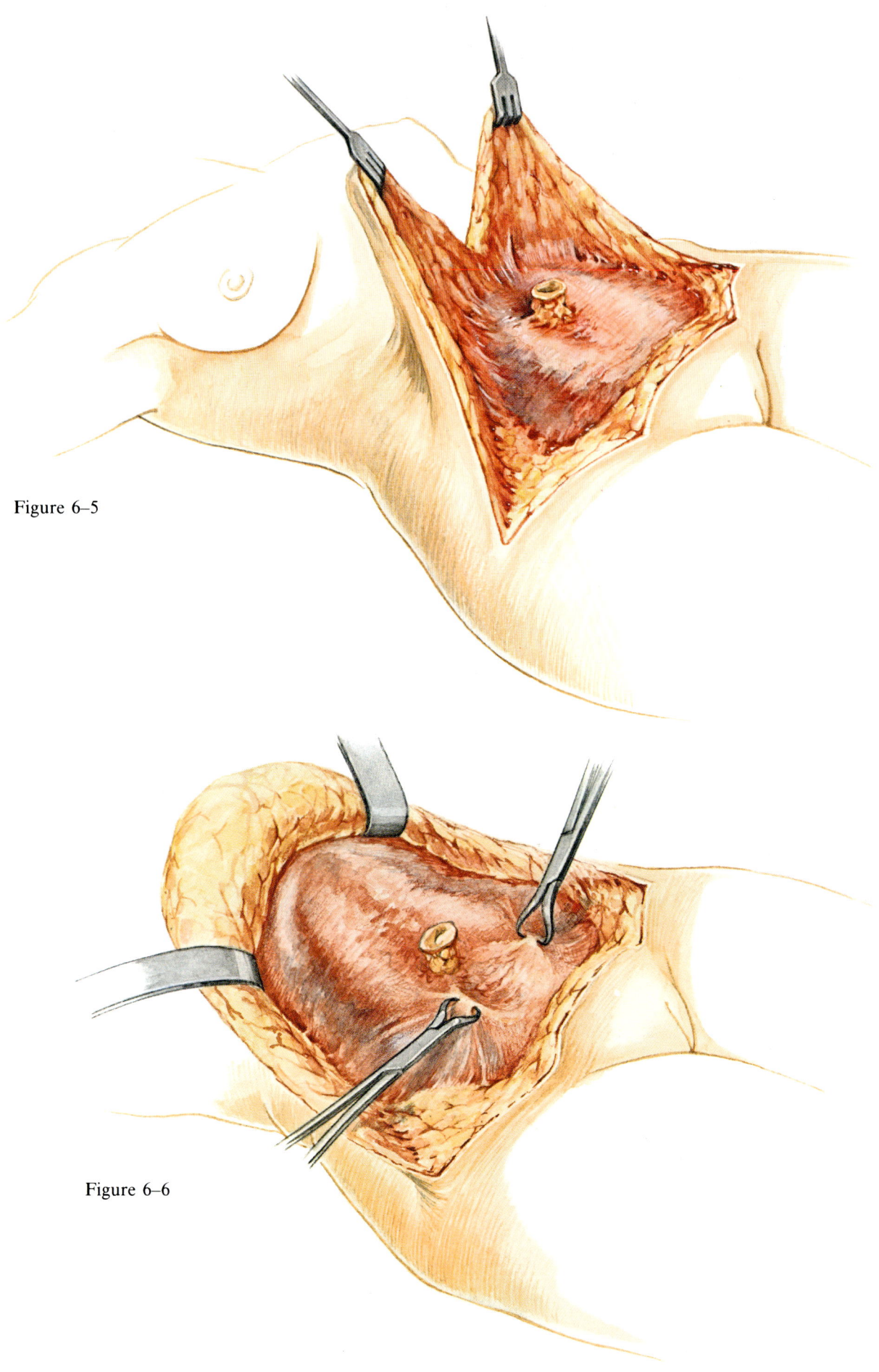

Figure 6–5

Figure 6–6

5. Continue dissection superior to the costal margin. For increased exposure during dissection, consider incising flap vertically in midline for a distance equal to the tissue to be removed (to the umbilicus as a rule). Most surgeons avoid vertical incisions superior to umbilicus (see Variations).
6. Secure hemostasis after abdominal flap is fully dissected.
7. Begin plication of rectus abdominus fascia (Fig. 6–6). Use wide figure-of-eight nonabsorbable suture (Figs. 6–7A and B, Fig. 6–8). Do not leave gaps in midline fascia repair especially near umbilicus (Fig. 6–9).

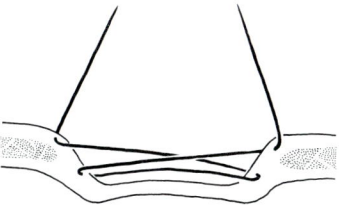
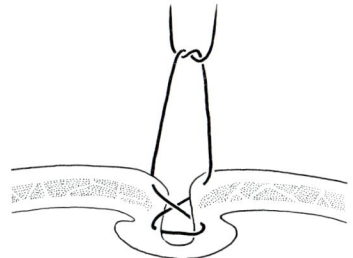

Figure 6–7

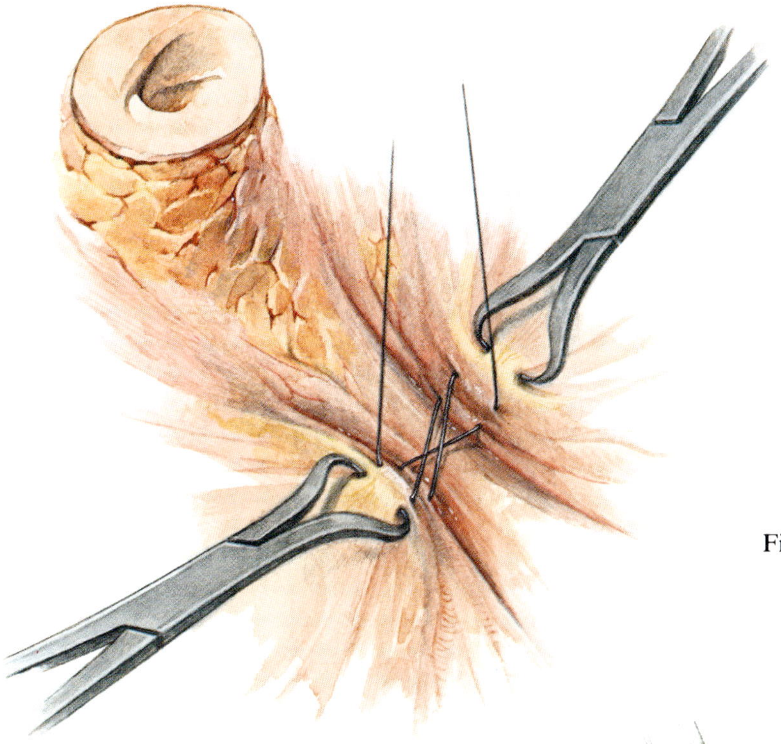

Figure 6–8

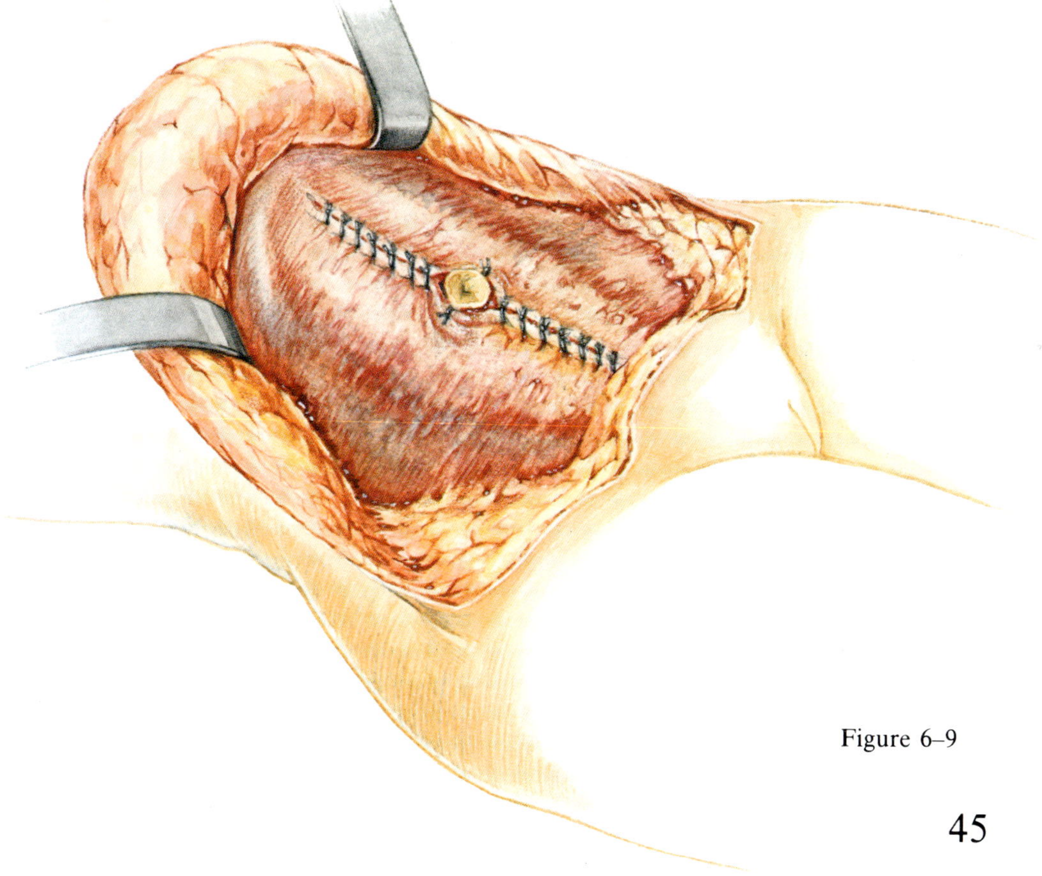

Figure 6–9

Abdominoplasty

8. Raise flap, irrigate wound, look carefully for bleeders, and coagulate each and every one. Also remove loose fat without adequate blood supply.
9. Now draw the abdominal flap downward (Fig. 6–10). Flex table more if needed to facilitate wound approximation. Identify new umbilical site. Make a curved incision. Depending on subcutaneous thickness, defatting around the new umbilical site may be necessary (Fig. 6–11).
10. Take one final look inside flap to make certain of hemostasis before beginning wound closure. Using towel clips or Kocher clamps draw abdominal flap inferiorly. Because the flap has been incised in midline, make certain that traction on each half is symmetric. Mark skin at line of intended excision. Avoid excess traction at this point.
11. Remove extra skin at this point; then thin flap, removing loose or overhanding fat. Achieve hemostasis of new flap margin. Upper flap should be thinned sufficiently for a beveled overlapping closure (Fig. 6–12).

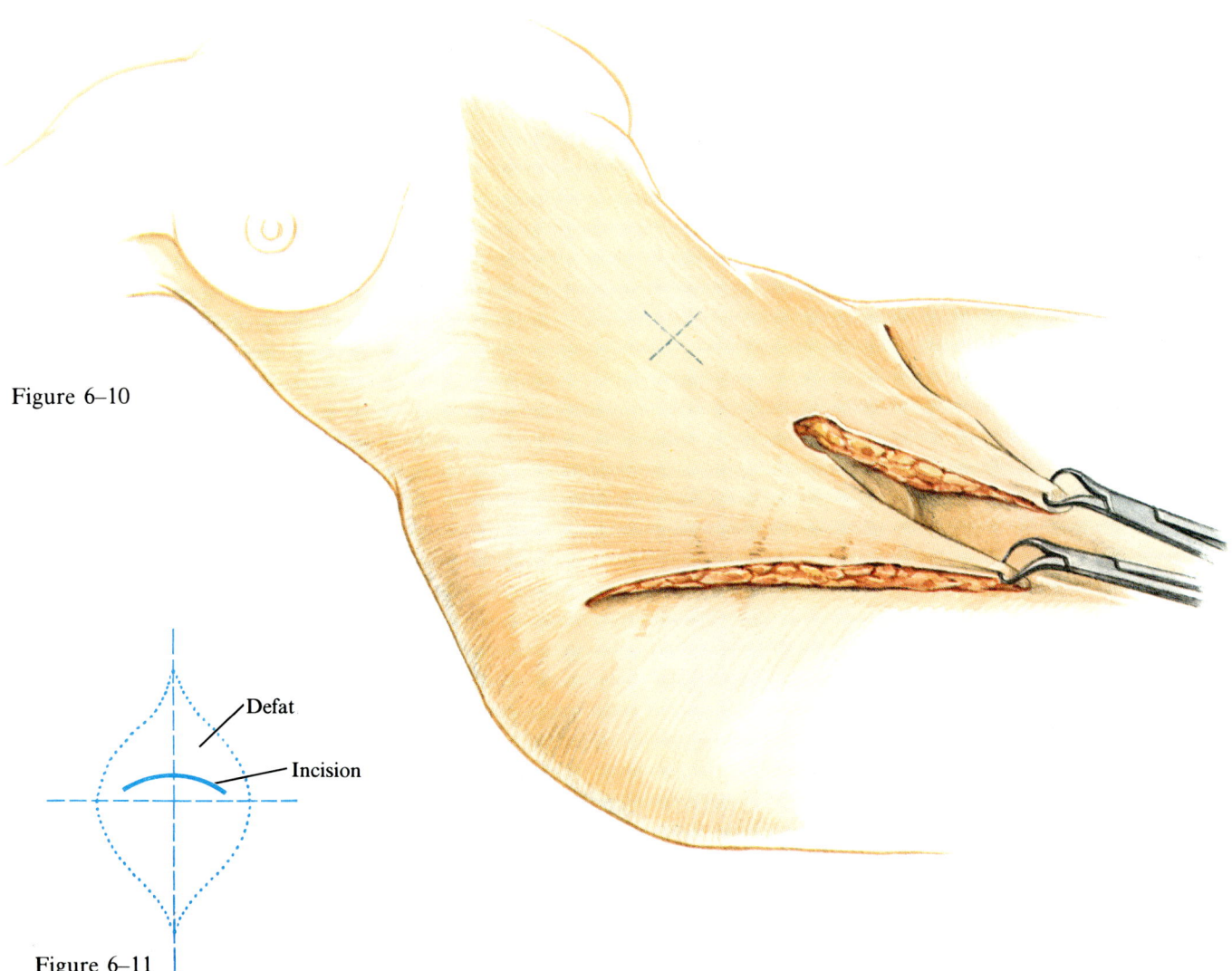

Figure 6–10

Figure 6–11

12. Place suction drains. Bring them out of each end of wound, not through a separate stab wound. Stab wounds leave unnecessary extra scars and may result in ischemic wound edges.
13. Deep closure is with heavy (2–0 or 3–0) absorbable sutures (Dexon® or Vicryl®). Place a few sutures in midline. Then close from lateral to medial, advancing abdominal flap with each stitch so as to avoid dogears or unnecessary lengthening of incision to eliminate dogears.
14. Close skin with running subcuticular Prolene® pullout suture. Start a new pullout every 8–10 cm. You will never be able to remove a single or even a double suture from a wound that long! Reinforce skin approximation with adhesive strips.
15. Complete approximation of umbilical skin to new opening in abdominal skin, taking skin border to underlying fascia (see Figs. 6–13 and 6–14).

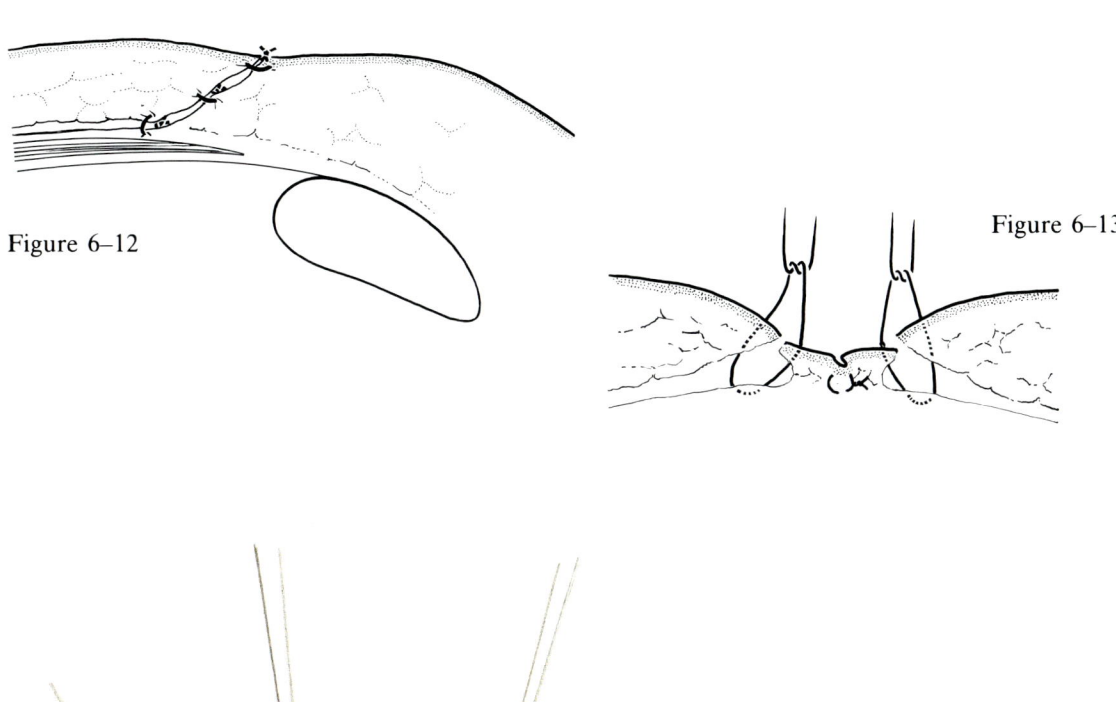

Figure 6–12

Figure 6–13

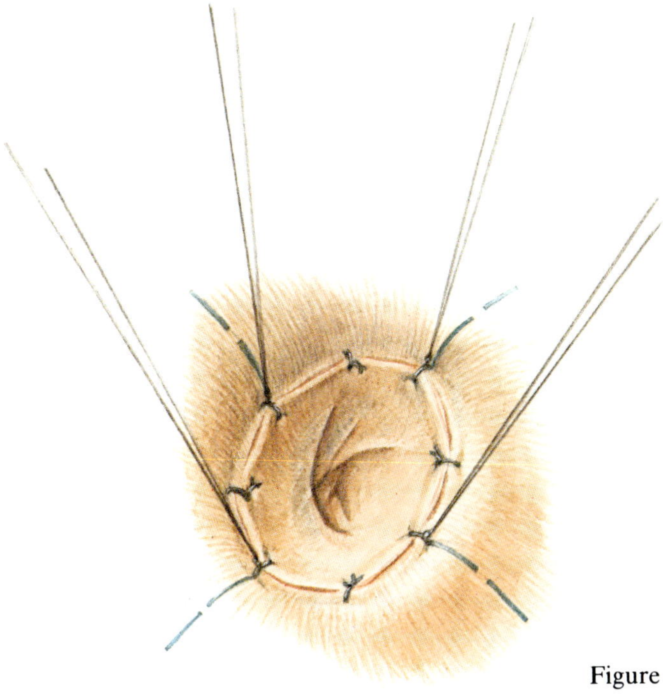

Figure 6–14

Figure 6–15

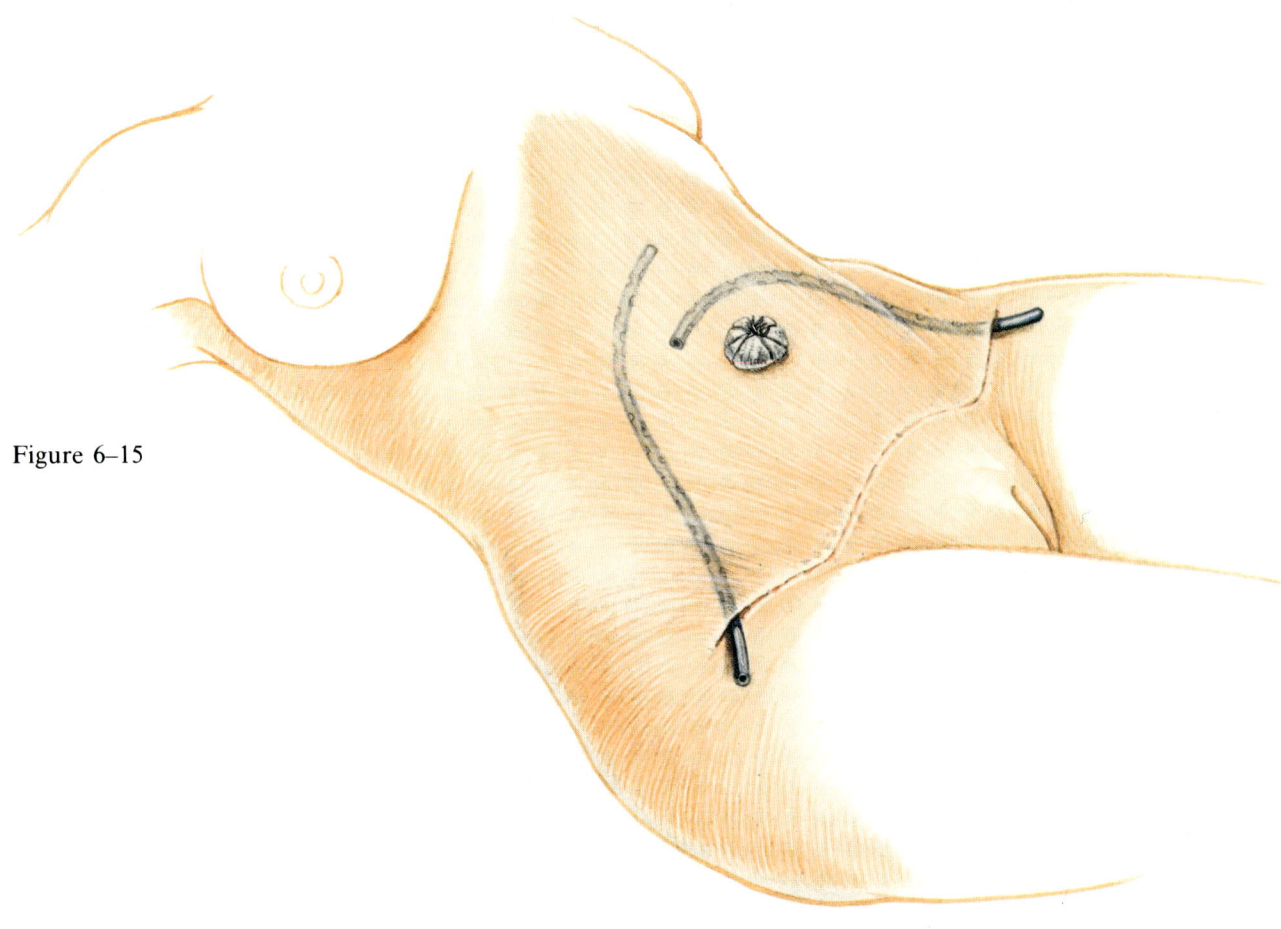

16. A circumferential dressing that provides meld compression is now applied (Fig. 6–15). Transfer patient to flexed bed in operating room. Recovery involves bedrest for 3–4 days, with brief standing on second day. Ambulation begins slowly.

Variations

Choice of Incisions
A variety of designs have been applied to provide a lower abdominal scar acceptable to most patients. Whereas many surgeons prefer a simple straight-line scar, others have popularized the W-shaped incision. Sharlply irregular scars tend to call attention to themselves. Each surgeon must select his own policy, it is hoped based on patient opinion and acceptance.

Excise Redundant Skin Ellipse First, Then Dissect Upper Abdominal Skin Flap
After developing confidence with abdominoplasty, beginning surgeons should consider initially excising the entire infraumbilical ellipse of redundant skin. Dissection of the upper abdominal flap then proceeds with greater ease because exposure is better. Adoption of this sequence requires that the surgeon be confident of wound approximation prior to flap immobilization. This is possible only when patients are screened carefully for surgery.

Electrocautery versus Knife Dissection

Opinions vary regarding whether knife or electrocautery dissection is preferable. Surgeons experienced with a knife say they can move just as quickly. Others say electrocautery is faster, and blood loss is diminished by immediate coagulation of vessels as the flap is dissected free. Either way, the larger perforating vessels of the abdominal wall must be clamped, divided, and ligated or coagulated.

Additional Reading

Regnault PCL. The history of abdominal dermolipectomy. Aesth Plast Surg 2:113–123, 1978. (Includes references from Kelly [1859] to Callia [1965]).

Guerrero-Santos J. Some problems and solutions in abdominoplasty. Aesth Plast Surg 4:227, 1980.

Grazer FM and Goldwyn RM. Abdominoplasty assessed by surgery with emphasis on complications. Plast Reconstr Surg 59:513, 1977.

Hunter GR, Crapo RO, Broadbent TR, Woolf RM. Pulmonary complications following abdominal lipectomy. Plast Reconstr Surg 71:809–813, 1983.

Guerrerosantos J, Dicksheet S, Carrillo C, Sandoval M. Umbilical reconstruction with secondary abdominoplasty. Ann Plast Surg 5:139–144, 1980.

Blepharoplasty

Carson M. Lewis and Leonard W. Glass

Background

European surgeons described excessive eyelid skin during the 19th century. Procedures for removal of redundant eyelid skin were reported early in the 20th century. Bourguet introduced eyelid fat removal in 1929 and it thereafter became an integral part of blepharoplasty. Castanares defined the compartments of eyelid fat and further refined blepharoplasty into the procedure we know today. Use of the skin-muscle flap was introduced by McIndoe. More recently, pretarsal fixation and other variations are a product of the ingenuity of Flowers and Sheen; orbicularis excision was popularized by Baker.

Indications

1. Excess eyelid skin (Fig. 7–1)
2. Prominent periorbital fat pads
3. Shallow or absent palpebral fold
4. Hypertrophic orbicularis muscle.

Contraindications

1. Too little skin
2. Diminished lower eyelid tone
3. Decreased tear production
4. Patient wants only removal of "crow's feet"

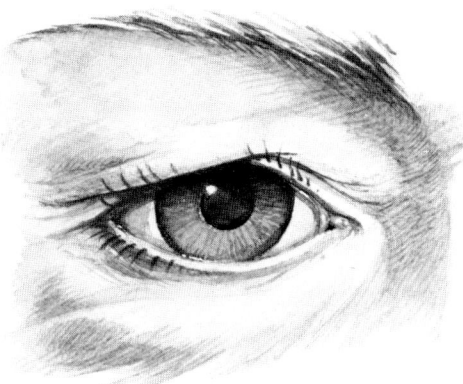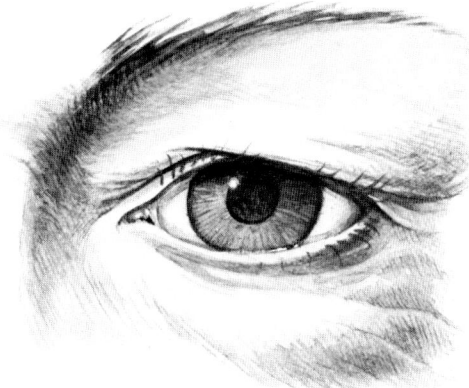

Figure 7–1

Blepharoplasty

5. Inability to close eye fully
6. Certain ocular diseases
7. Brow ptosis without excessive eyelid skin
8. Epiphora.

What the Patient Needs to Know Before Surgery

Will Occur

1. Periorbital swelling and ecchymosis
2. Scars (lateral portion remains conspicuous longer than medial eyelid scar)

Can Occur

1. Subconjunctival hemorrhage
2. Conjunctivitis
3. Diminished tear production (dry eye syndrome)
4. Hematoma
5. Temporary visual blurring
6. Epiphora
7. Ectropion
8. Persistent discoloration of lower eyelid skin
9. Blindness (rare but it has been reported).

What the Surgeon Must Know

The orbicularis oculi muscle encircles the eye (Fig. 7–2), is anchored medially to the lacrimal crest, and laterally to the orbital wall by way of the respective canthal ligaments. The thin eyelid skin is firmly adherent to this muscle. Beneath the muscle lies the septum orbitale, a membrane responsible for restraining the periorbital fat, albeit less successfully as age advances.

The orbital fat is held in compartments, two above and three below. The most medial compartments in each lid contain white fat; lateral compartments hold yellow fat. The physiologic basis for this anatomic distinction is not understood. The lacrimal gland lies lateral to both fat pads in the upper eyelid and may be ptotic. The lacrimal collecting system is entirely medial to the lower lid punctum. Skin incisions lateral to the punctum will not disturb drainage of tears.

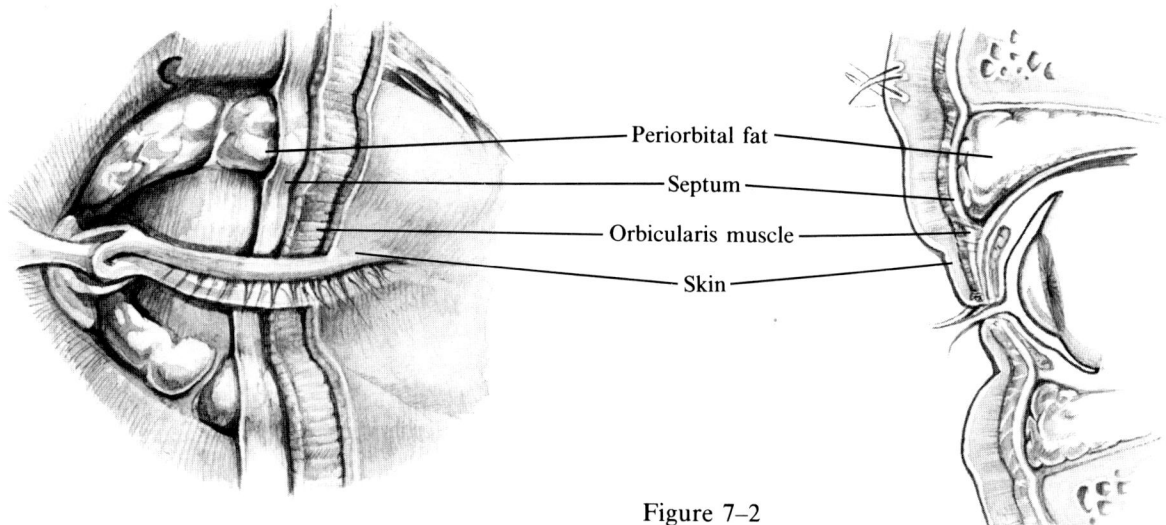

Figure 7–2

Operative Planning

The palpebral fold of the upper lid is the result of adherence of the skin to the levator palpebra superioris muscle. This adherence is absent in Orientals.

The depth of the bony orbit varies widely. In the presence of proptosis, removal of the periorbital fat may exaggerate ocular prominence.

Operative Planning

Begin with a thorough and fully documented preoperative evaluation. Include determination of vision, levator function, tear production, lower lid tone, and any asymmetry of eyelid form or function. Finally, assess skin surplus. Note presence of ptosis, muscle hypertrophy, and location and severity of fat proptosis.

Blepharoplasty begins with a careful marking of the skin with the patient sitting upright. Elevate the brow and mark the proposed site of the upper palpebral crease, a curved line, 8–10 mm from the lash line in midline; less distant at either end (Fig. 7–3). This line should also extend beyond the lateral canthus. The upper lid ellipse is completed by selecting the upper border of skin to be removed. Fold excess skin between thumb and index finger to facilitate this judgement (Fig. 7–4).

The lower lid incision is placed 2–3 mm beneath the lid margin, perhaps in a natural crease, extending from beneath punctum medially to the lateral extent of the lower lid, extending laterally into the skin crease 1–1.5 cm beyond the canthus (Fig. 7–5). Press on globe and mark location of fat pads. Also mark level of the inferior orbital rim.

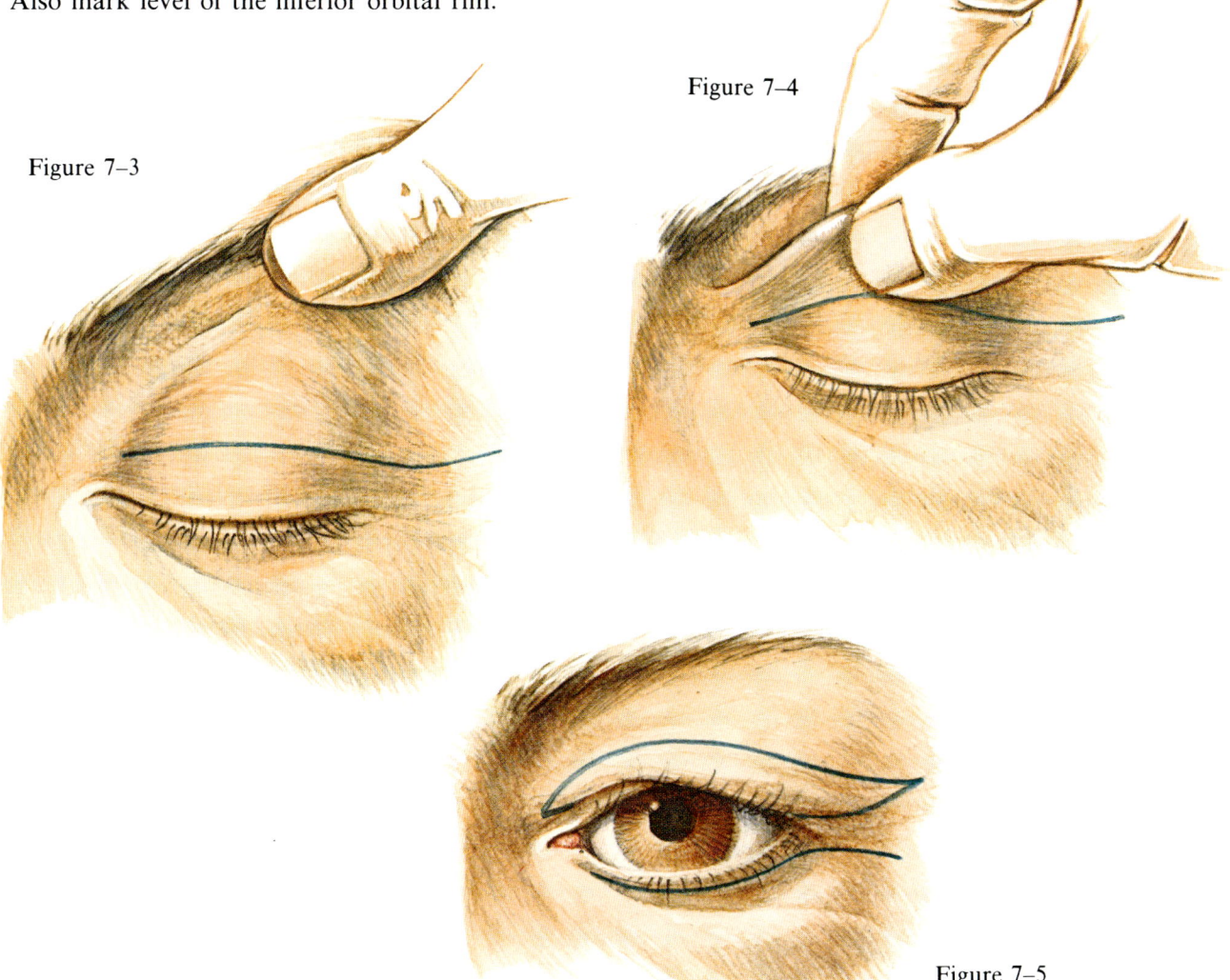

Figure 7–3

Figure 7–4

Figure 7–5

Blepharoplasty

Regional Anesthesia

1. Use 1–2% xylocaine with epinephrine (1:100,000 or 1:200,000). Inject via 27-gauge needle.
2. Inject from lateral position, tangential to lid surface, always directing the point away from the globe. **NEVER** point needle toward the globe. A sudden movement by the patient could result in tragedy.
3. Infiltrate the entire field of dissection, but with a small volume (no more than 2 cc for each lid).

Operative Techniques

Upper Eyelid

1. First incise the premarked skin ellipse (Fig. 7–6). Then remove skin, dissecting carefully on top of the orbicularis muscle (Fig. 7–7).
2. Divide fibers of the orbicularis just superior to the inferior wound margin. Lift muscle and identify fat pads beneath the septum orbitale (Fig. 7–8). Avoid injury to levator aponeurosis and tarsus lying deep to fat.
3. Do not miss the most medial fat pad. Remember, it will be pale white in color (Fig. 7–9).

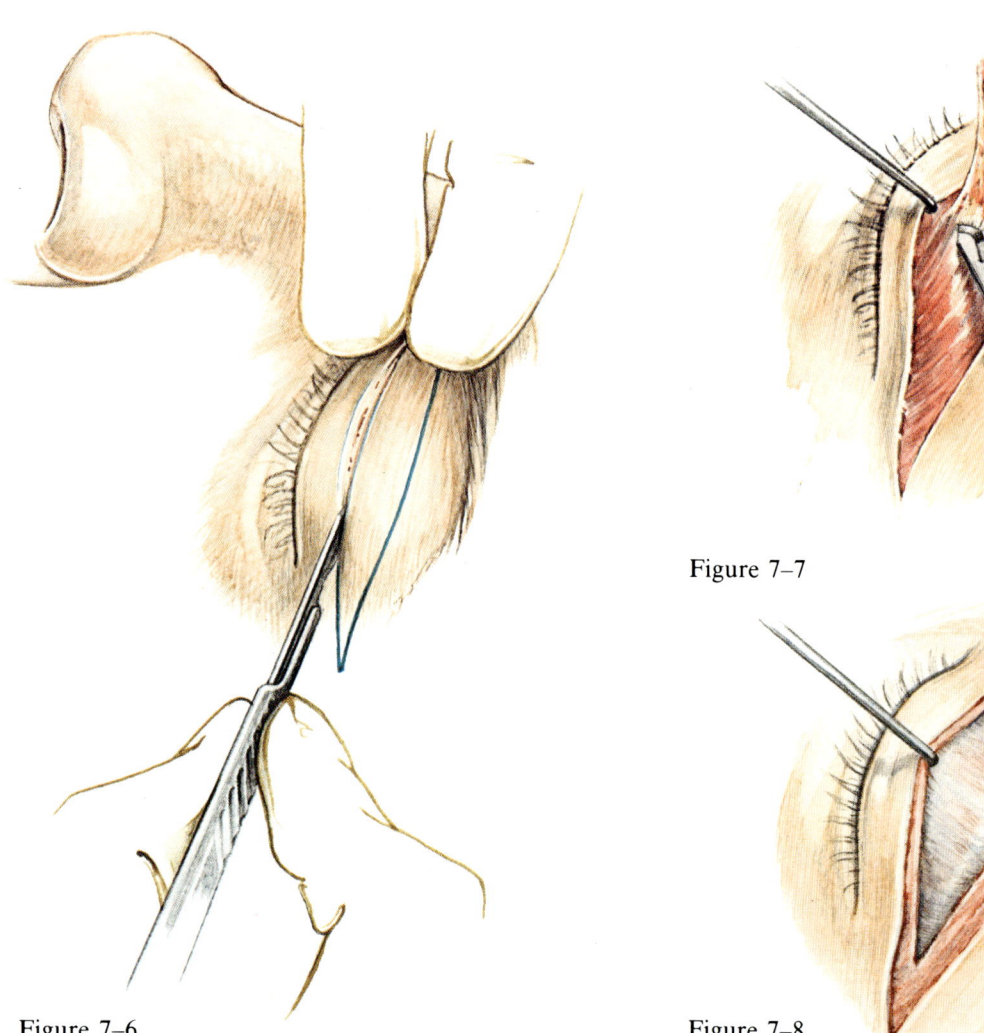

Figure 7–6

Figure 7–7

Figure 7–8

4. Microcoagulate each fat pad vessel as it is divided. No bleeding vessel should be permitted. Retract into the orbit.
5. If the lacrimal gland is ptotic, affix it to periosteum of lateral orbital wall with fine sutures.
6. Remove a thin strip of orbicularis muscle along the entire length of the eyelid (Fig. 7–10).
7. Secure hemostasis.
8. Either close the wound (running subcuticular sutures) or leave it open until lower lid is completed.

Lower Eyelid

1. Incise skin lateral to canthus. Insert Stephens tenotomy scissors just beneath skin, opening the remaining subciliary incision as marked without cutting lashes.
2. Protect the globe by inserting traction suture in the upper wound margin, attach mosquito clamp, and drape it over forehead gently.
3. a. *Skin Flap Technique:* Dissect skin only from underlying muscle to level of orbital rim (Fig. 7–11).
   b. *Skin/Muscle Flap Technique:* Incise skin and elevate lower flap a short distance. Then enter muscle, dividing it along a line parallel to fibers, eventually reaching orbital rim.

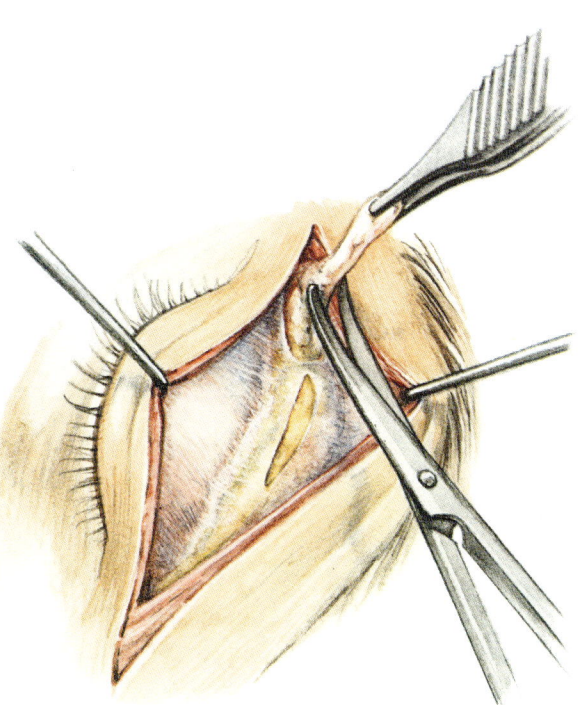

Figure 7–9

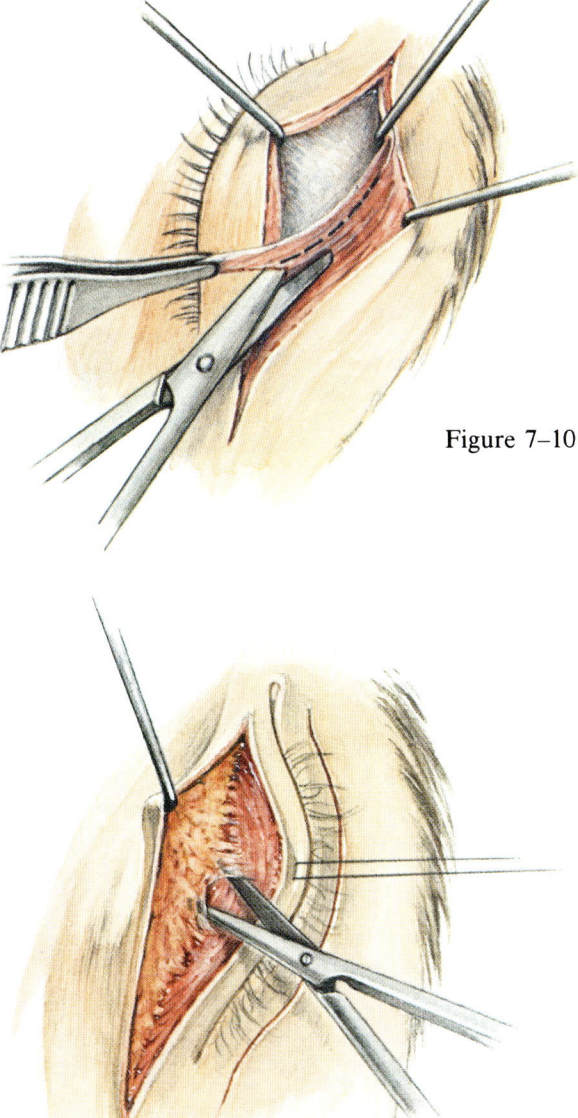

Figure 7–10

Figure 7–11

Blepharoplasty

Figure 7–12

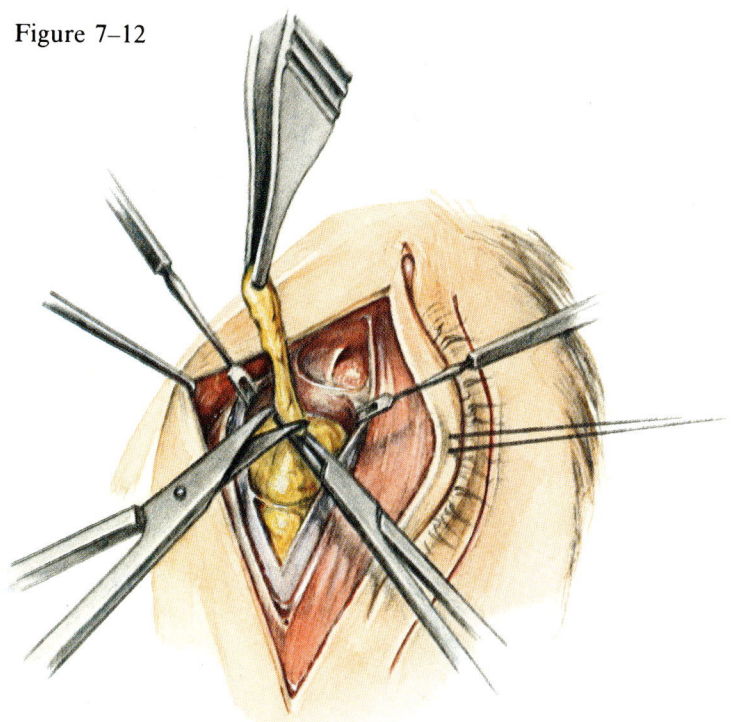

Figure 7–13

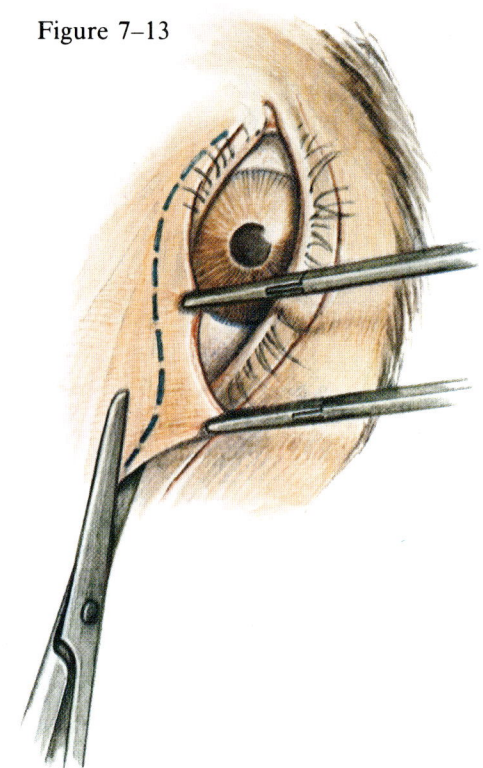

4. Open septum orbitale, and identify each of three fat compartments. Remove fat by pulling gently (patient may feel this); coagulate visible vessels, then divide pedicle. Surgeons often clamp fat pedicle before dividing—then coagulate (Fig. 7–12).
5. Establish hemostasis.
6. Trim excess skin from the lower eyelid, not to an excess or ectropion will result (Fig. 7–13).
7. Close upper eyelid incision, check for hemostasis again, then close lower eyelid excision.
8. Apply iced sponges in recovery room or later at home. Send patient home without blindfold. Instruct patient to cleanse suture lines with Q-tips and dilute peroxide.

Variations

Orbicularis Muscle Hyperplasia
In the presence of excess muscle of lower eyelid, a small amount can be excised from the lower edge of the incision. Whenever muscle is to be removed, develop a skin–muscle flap.

Avoiding Ectropion
Many suggestions are advocated such as opening mouth before marking lower lid excess. When lower eyelid muscle tone is deficient, consider wedge excision and tightening of lower lid (Kundt-Zymanowsi procedure) at time of blepharoplasty.

Correcting Lateral Brow Prominence
This problem can be solved by reattaching lacrimal gland, or in extreme cases, exposing orbital rim and reducing bony prominence.

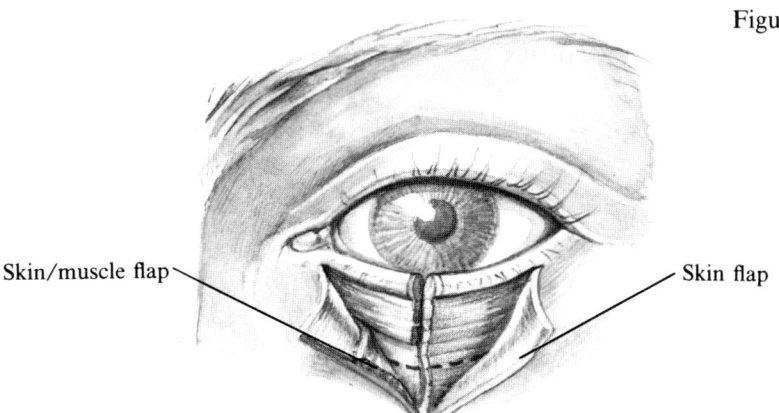

Figure 7–14

Issues

Skin/Muscle Flap versus Skin Flap (Fig. 7–14)
This is probably a variation but many surgeons try to make it an issue. Those who select the skin flap technique consider the problem to be largely redundant skin and do not wish to create downward traction of eyelid by adherent orbicularis fibers. Those who use the skin muscle flap desire more direct access to fat pads, or they plan to resect hyperplastic muscle along with skin, or they plan a very conservative skin excision. Versatile surgeons use both techniques depending on circumstance.

Rotate Lateral? Rotate Medial?
After freeing redundant lower eyelid tissues some advocate lateral rotation of skin at the time of closure; others are convinced that medial rotation is preferable.

Creation of Upper Palpebral Crease
Some advocate pretarsal fixation of skin to the underlying levator aponeurosis (Sheen); others declare excision of a levator strip sufficient to create zone of contraction during healing that will ensure a fold (Baker).

Browlift at Time of Blepharoplasty (or Vice-Versa)
Conservative surgeons avoid combining the procedures out of fear that overresection may occur. Others insist that with judgement, browlift can be combined with blepharoplasty, *in that order.* Judge extent of upper lid skin excision only after browlift is complete.

Additional Reading

Stephenson KL. The history of blepharoplasty to correct blepharochalasis. Aesth Plast Surg 1:177–194, 1977. (A definitive and thorough historical analysis.)

Castanares S. Blepharoplasty for herniated intraorbital fat—anatomical basis for a new approach. Plast Reconstr Surg 8:46, 1951. (A classic description of the principles we apply today.)

Castanares S. Ectropion after blepharoplasty. Prevention and treatment. Aesth Plast Surg 2:125–140, 1978. (An important discussion of the most feared complications of blepharoplasty.)

Sheen JH. A change in the technique of supratarsal fixation in upper blepharoplasty. Plast Reconstr Surg 59(6):831–834, 1977.

Sheen JH. Tarsal fixation in lower blepharoplasty. Plast Reconstr Surg 62(1):24–31, 1978.

Baker TJ, Gordon HL, and Mosienko P. Upper lid blepharoplasty. Plast Reconst Surg 60:692, 1977.

Rees TD and Dupuis C. Baggy eyelids in young adults. Plast Reconst Surg 43:381, 1969.

Rees TD. Correction of ectropion resulting from blepharoplasty. Plast Reconst Surg 50:1, 1972.

Rees TD. The "dry eye" complication after blepharoplasty. Plast Reconst Surg 56:375, 1975.

Facelift

Matthew Gleason and Jose Guerrerosantos

Background

The origins of facelifting are obscure. Early practitioners of the art were unwilling to record their experience. Perhaps they were embarrassed to let their colleagues know what they were doing; perhaps they were too selfish to share their knowledge.

Historians of cosmetic surgery assign credit for the first facelift to Lexer in 1906. Joseph claimed precedent in 1921 for a facelift he had done in 1912. Few if any care who was first. All that counts is that by 1930, facelifting was an established procedure practiced by surgeons in many cities: Passot in Paris, Stern in Vienna, Hunt in New York, Booth in Seattle, Bames in Los Angeles. All early facelifts were characterized by limited undermining.

Our most respected forefathers, Gillies, Blair, Ferris-Smith, and many others became proficient with facelifting. Yet, they did not formally describe their techniques or record their results.

Not until the 1960s were aesthetic surgeons secure enough and sufficiently proud of their work to inform their colleagues of such advances as parotid plication (Pangman), or the total circumferential incision (Gonzalez-Ulloa). The bold suggestions of these and other surgeons' writing nearly two decades ago were not widely applied until recently.

The refinements of more recent surgeons will be referred to in this chapter.

Indications

1. Aging deformity (Fig. 8–1)
2. Unilateral facial paralysis.

Contraindications

1. Skin not loose enough
2. Skin not suitable for surgery
   a. Heavy, oily skin with thick subcutaneous tissues ("fat face")
   b. Actinic damage to skin with deep creases and inelastic skin (in this case consider chemical peel).
   c. History of connective tissue disease, e.g. scleroderma, Raynaud's phenomenon, etc.
   d. Prior irradiation.

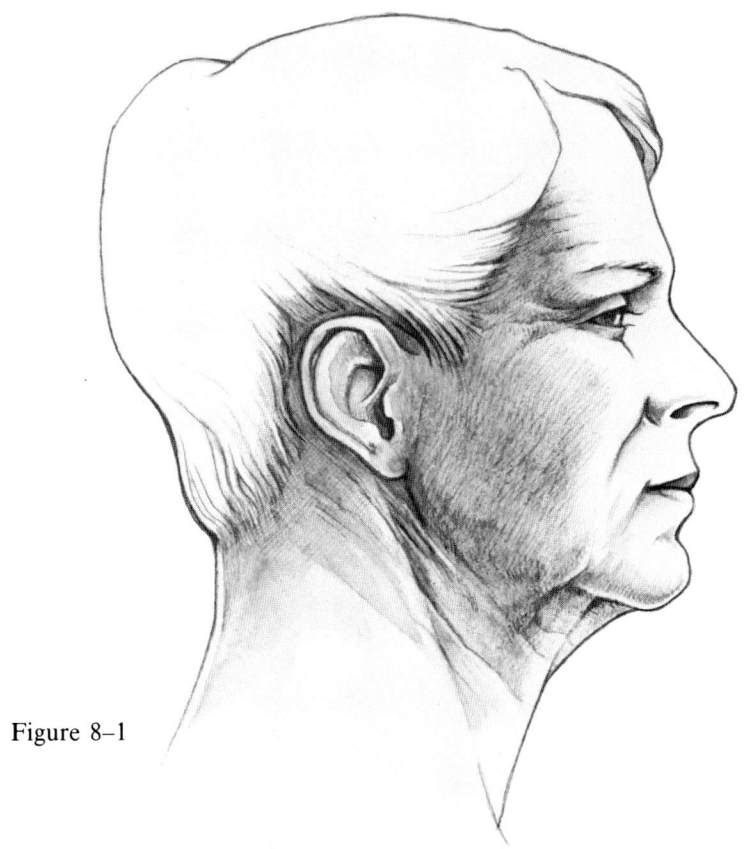

Figure 8–1

3. Systemic illnesses such as uncompensated heart disease or previous heart surgery, labile hypertension, cortisone therapy, etc.
4. Unrealistic expectation
5. Patient reluctant to accept surgical scars
6. Strong opposition to surgery by spouse, children, or friends
7. Acute or chronic emotional depression (postpone until therapy is given).

What the Patient Needs to Know Before Surgery

Will Occur

1. Surgical scars
2. Edema and ecchymosis for several weeks after surgery
3. Improvement, *not miraculous rejuvenation*
4. Minimal correction of lower neck wrinkles, acne scars, or deep nasolabial folds. Forehead furrows, eyelids, and perioral creases require separate procedures.
5. Short-term depression and disappointment. Patients should be warned that any surgery, including cosmetic surgery, is a stress to the system and that stress is experienced as "depression." Tell patients that it is normal to be depressed.

Can Occur

1. Hematoma (fewer than 5% incidence)
2. Loss of skin sensation for several months
3. Injury to facial nerves (mandibular, frontal, or buccal)
4. Skin necrosis (especially behind the ears)
5. Long-lasting edema

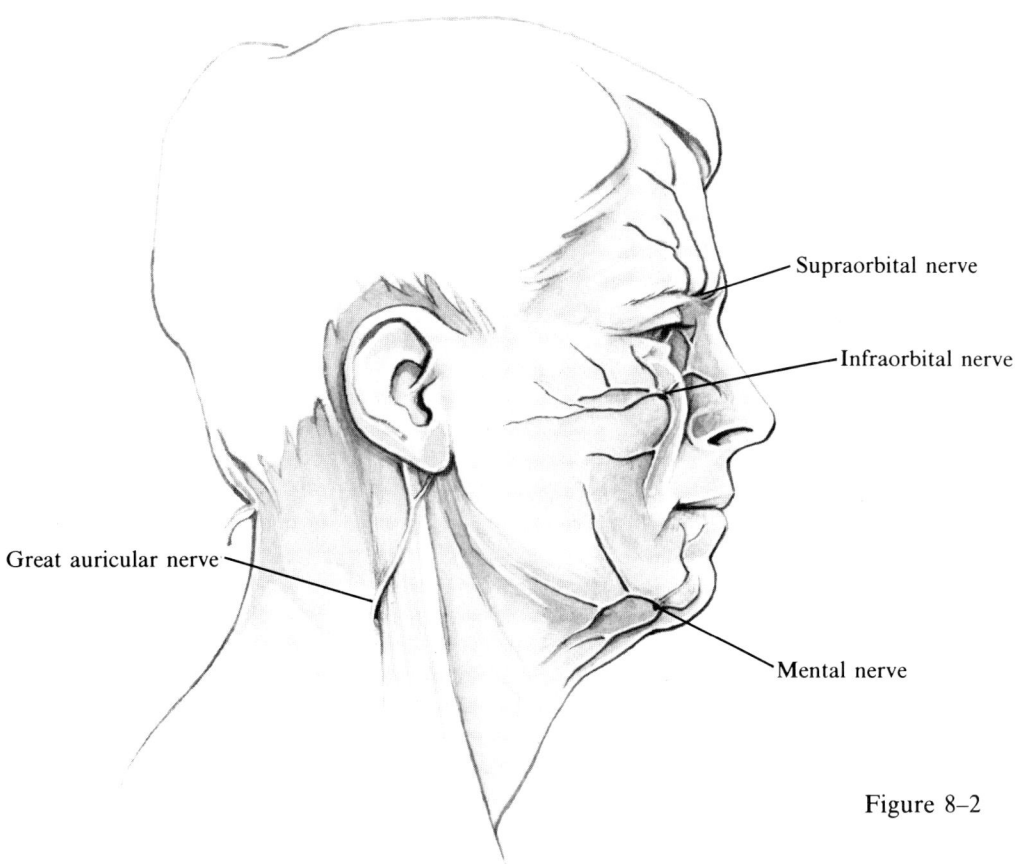

Figure 8-2

6. Hypertrophy of scars behind ears and neck
7. Change of hairline in temple and neck
8. Alopecia—normally temporary, occasionally permanent.

What the Surgeon Must Know

1. The hair-bearing skin of the temple is thick, the follicles deep, and the subcutaneous fat sparse. The veins are large and they bleed freely. The skin anterior to the ear is thin and the subcutaneous fat layer generous. The skin behind the ear is thin with little subcutaneous fat; tension can therefore result in skin necrosis. The lateral neck skin is adherent to the sternocleidomastoid muscle. The posterior neck skin is thick and well-vascularized.
2. The temporal scalp is elevated easily from the temporalis fascia. The frontalis branch of the facial nerve (VII) becomes superficial near the lateral orbit.
3. The cheek skin is easily elevated from the superficial muscular aponeurotic system (SMAS) which overlays the parotid gland. The fibrous malar fat is not easily undermined. Bleeding is brisk near the nasolabial fold where motor nerves become superficial.
4. The thick neck skin posterior to the sternocleidomastoid muscle can be dissected with ease, but dissection over the sternocleidomastoid sheath is difficult because of fibrous skin attachments. The great auricular nerve can be injured if the sheath is entered. Anterior to the sternocleidomastoid muscle, the dissection proceeds with ease in the soft subcutaneous fat between skin and the platysma muscle.
5. The trigeminal nerve (V) provides sensation to the skin of the face (Fig. 8–2). The ophthalmic nerve (V_1) leaves the cranium via the supraorbital

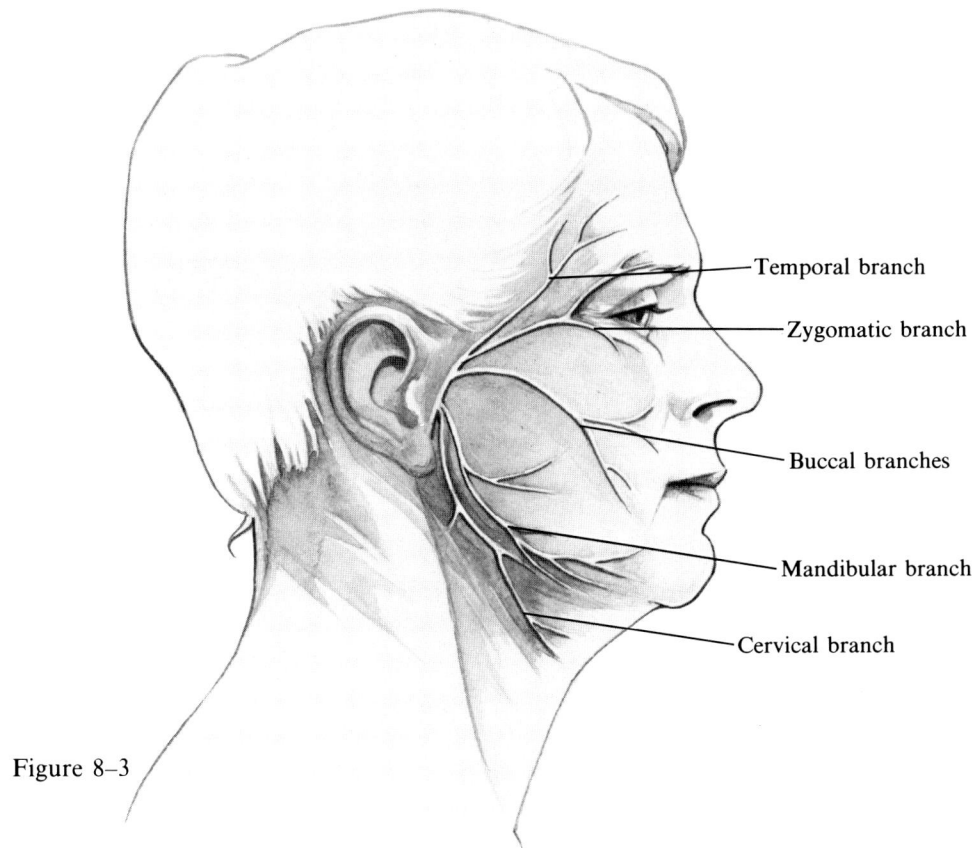

Figure 8–3

fissure in the medial one-third of superior orbital margin. It is sensory to the skin of the forehead, upper lid, nose, upper eyelid, and periosteum of the orbit. The maxillary nerve (V_2) exits via the infraorbital foramen and innervates the face, lower eyelids, buccal mucous membranes, gums, and upper teeth. The mandibular nerve (V_3) exits the mandibular foramen and provides sensation to the lower teeth, the skin of the lower jaw, side of the head, auricle, and temporal mandibular joint. The great auricular nerve (C2,3) is the largest ascending branch of the cervical plexus. It rounds the posterior border of the sternocleidomastoid, passes deep to the platysma, and accompanies the external jugular vein toward the angle of the jaw where it divides: an anterior branch to the skin of the lower lower auricle and a posterior branch supplying the scalp behind the ear.

6. The facial nerve (VII) is motor to the face (Fig. 8–3). There are five branches that the plastic surgeon should be aware of. They are arranged like the fingers of the hand.
   a. The thumb represents the temporal branch which crosses the zygomatic arch deep to the temporal fascia to innervate the frontalis muscle. This nerve is easily injured during a facelift.
   b. The index finger represents the zygomatic branch. It crosses the zygomatic bone to supply the muscles of the upper lip.
   c. The middle finger represents the buccal branches to the muscles of the upper lip. These are endangered during elevation of the SMAS.
   d. The ring finger is analogous to the mandibular branch. It crosses the mandible, deep to the platysma, and supplies the lower lip and chin. It can be injured during the platysma dissection.
   e. The little finger represents the cervical branch which passes below the mandibular angle deep to the platysma, which it innervates.

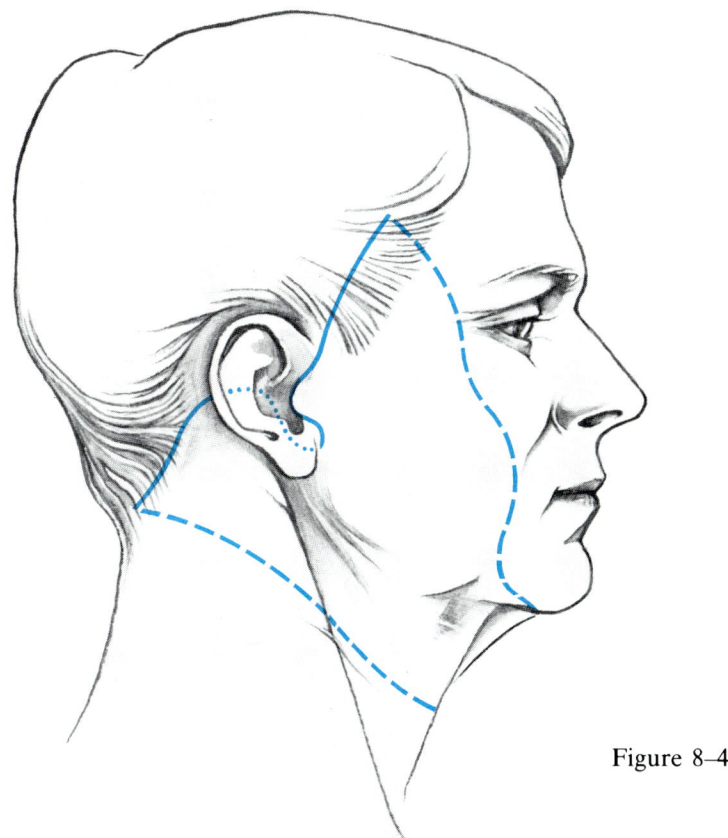

Figure 8–4

The most commonly encountered postoperative facial paralysis is temporary and is produced by the local anesthetic. All plastic surgeons have passed anxious moments awaiting nerve recovery. If paralysis persists for 48 h, assume that a nerve has been damaged. Encourage the patient by telling her that distal nerve injuries are usually self-limited. (I employ faradic stimulation and frequent office visits to maintain morale, mine and theirs!). A pseudopalsy of the lower lip can follow division of the platysma at too high a level. The platysma serves as an anchor to the depressor muscles of the lip. Function returns to normal as the platysma reattaches itself. Every surgeon performing facelift surgery should know the branches of the facial nerve as well as he knows his own hand (Pitanguy; Dingman).

7. The blood supply to the face is generous. This fact explains why infections are rare and hematomas are frequent. A vessel commonly cut is the superficial temporal vein, which may not bleed until after surgery. Branches of the superficial temporal artery are not often a postoperative problem because prompt bleeding catches the surgeon's eye. The malar fat tissue contains small vessels and requires meticulous hemostasis. In the neck, the external jugular vein can be injured, especially when the dissection is deeper than necessary.

Operative Design

Mark the patient while she/he sits upright (Fig. 8–4). The jowls, nasolabial folds, and platysma bands can be more easily identified. They will disappear after the patient lies down. Clip the temple and the neck hair lightly; do not shave. A curving methylene blue line is drawn high in the temporal hairline (at the level of the eyebrow) and continued vertically anterior to the ear. A small, horizontal "dart" can be made just above the tragus and the line continued in front of or behind the tragus (see Variations.) The line then curves around the earlobe. I prefer to make the postauricular markings directly in the sulcus rather than on the conchal skin because there is less bleeding. (In either case, the incision comes to lie in the sulcus.) When the level of the mastoid bone is reached, the marking traverses horizontally into the hair of the neck (see Variations). Other helpful markings include the nasolabial folds, the triangular shaped "jowls" (accumulation of submandibular fat), and vertical bands of platysma. The external jugular vein is also marked if seen.

Anesthesia

Sedate the patients very well prior to surgery. Begin an intravenous saline infusion and inject 10 mg of Valium in 2.5-mg increments. This permits for infiltration with local anesthesia without extraordinary discomfort. Use 0.5% xylocaine with epinephrine 1:200,000; your limit is 100 cc. Use a No. 25 spinal needle to minimize the volume injected. Inject both sides prior to draping so that deep sedation need be given only at the beginning of surgery. Manipulation of the longer spinal needle requires skill but minimizes numerous skin penetrations. Begin in the temple. Continue injecting anterior to the ear, above the zygoma, and lateral to the orbit. The second infiltration is in front of the tragus, into the remaining cheek and nasolabial fold. Place the third injection just below the angle of the mandible and fan out to include the lateral and anterior neck, as well as the sheath of sternocleidomastoid. The final injection is in the mastoid skin. From here, anesthetize the postauricular tissues and neck posterior to the sternomastoid. Occasionally, a separate injection is given along the midposterior border of the sternocleidomastoid muscle, further blocking the cervical plexus. Inject additional anesthetic as needed throughout surgery.

Operative Technique

Make the initial incision with a No. 15 blade as high up in the temporal hairline as the hair will allow. Continue your incision down in front of, around, and posterior to the ear; end in the lateral neck (Fig. 8–5). Elevate the skin of the tragus with a small two-pronged skin hook and with a No. 15 blade dissect the skin away from the tragal cartilage for several millimeters (Fig. 8–6). Begin the dissection in front of the ear and proceed superiorward, separating the thick temple skin and the hair follicles, from the glistening temporalis fascia (Fig. 8–7). Avoid injury to the large, superficial temporal veins you will encounter in this region. Use electrocautery frequently and carefully. If branches of the superficial temporal artery are divided, ligate them to prevent late hematoma formation.

Stop undermining as you enter the mobile fat near the nasolabial fold (Fig. 8–8). Dissecting further is of little benefit and the buccal branch of the facial nerve can be injured. Continue the dissection through the soft tissues over the mandible. Elevate the neck flap with a skin hook and note the ease with which the skin is dissected posterior to the sternocleidomastoid muscle. Dissection is difficult over the sternocleidomastoid because fibrous bands connect the sheath to the skin. If you enter the sheath, you will risk injury to the great auricular nerve. This nerve is large and easily repaired. Failure to repair it can result in a painful neuroma. Anterior to the sternocleidomastoid muscle, you may proceed with ease through the soft subcutaneous tissues to

Operative Technique

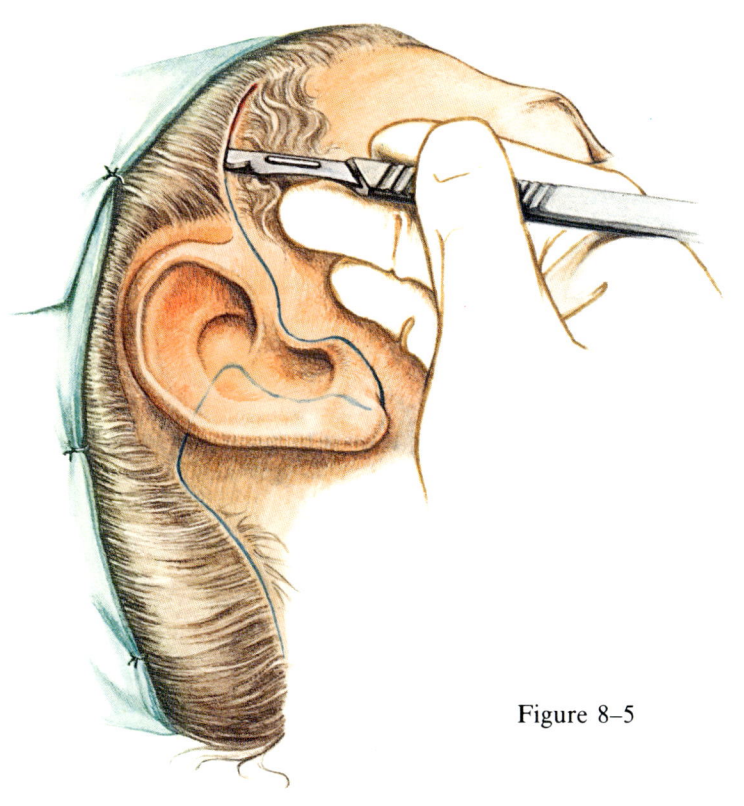

Figure 8–5

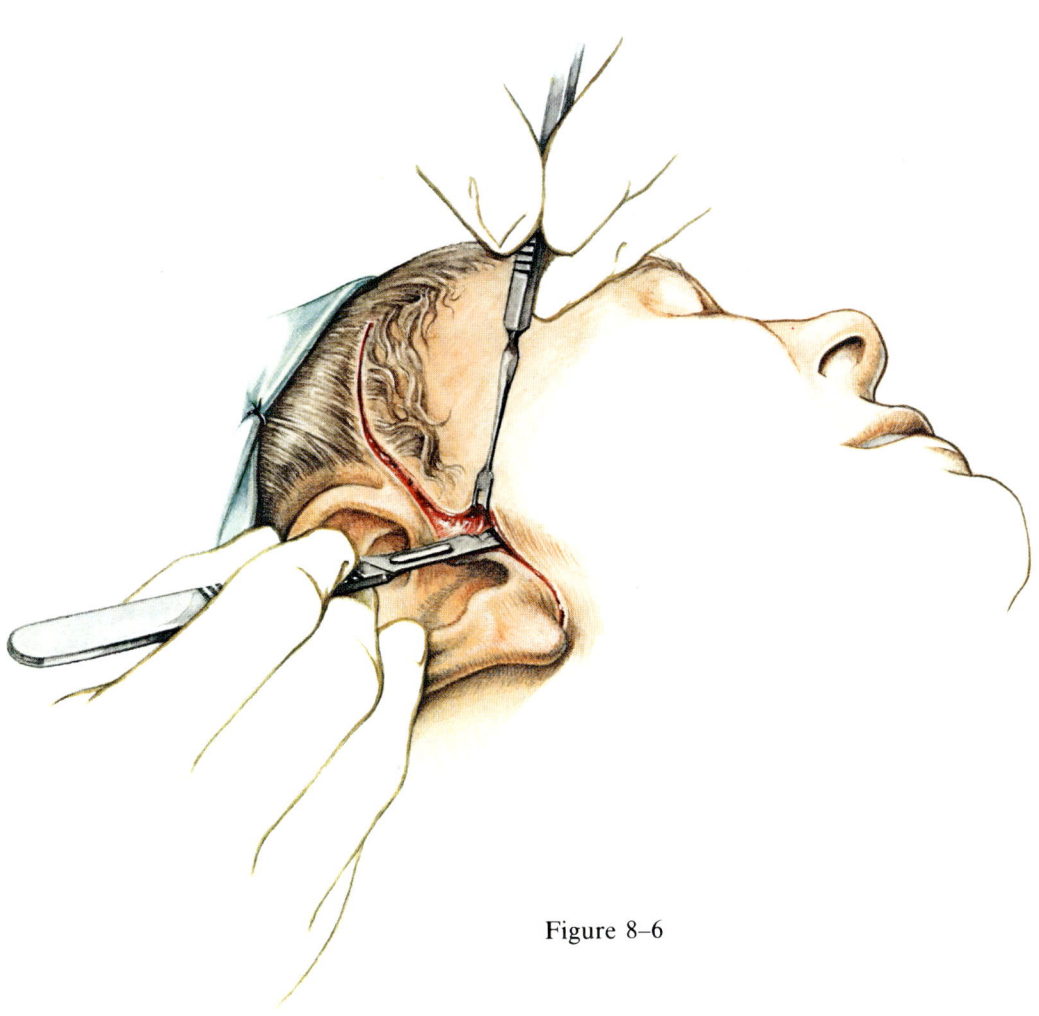

Figure 8–6

65

Facelift

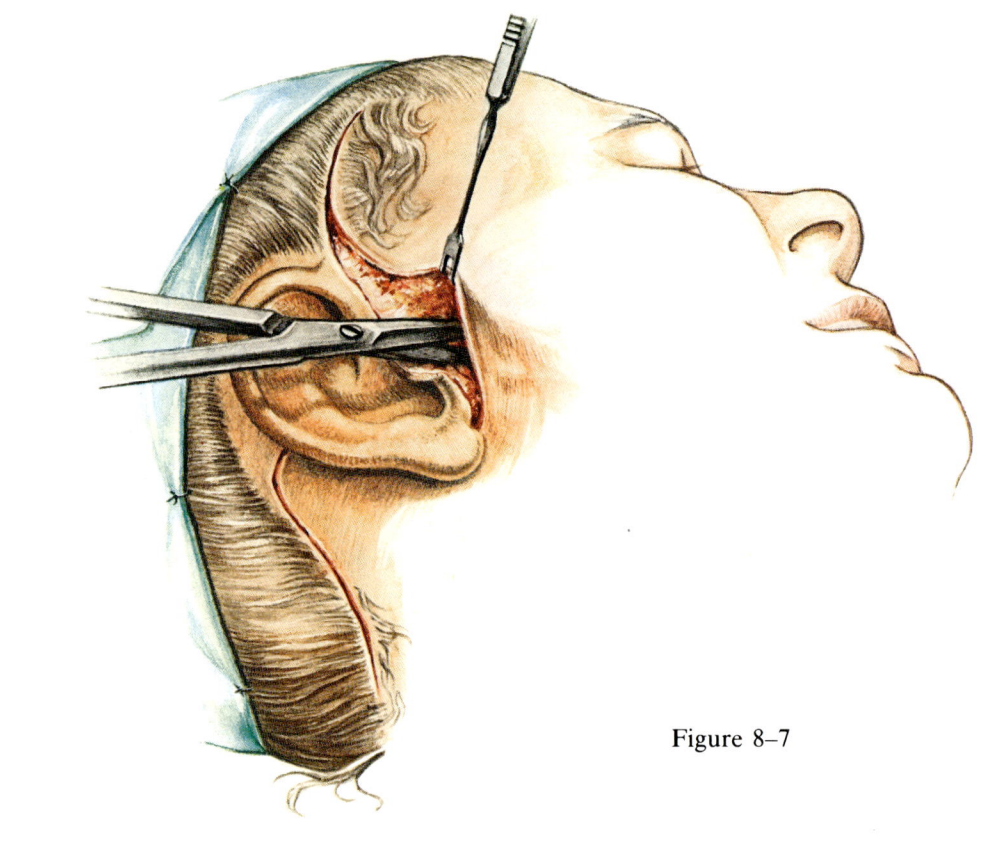

Figure 8–7

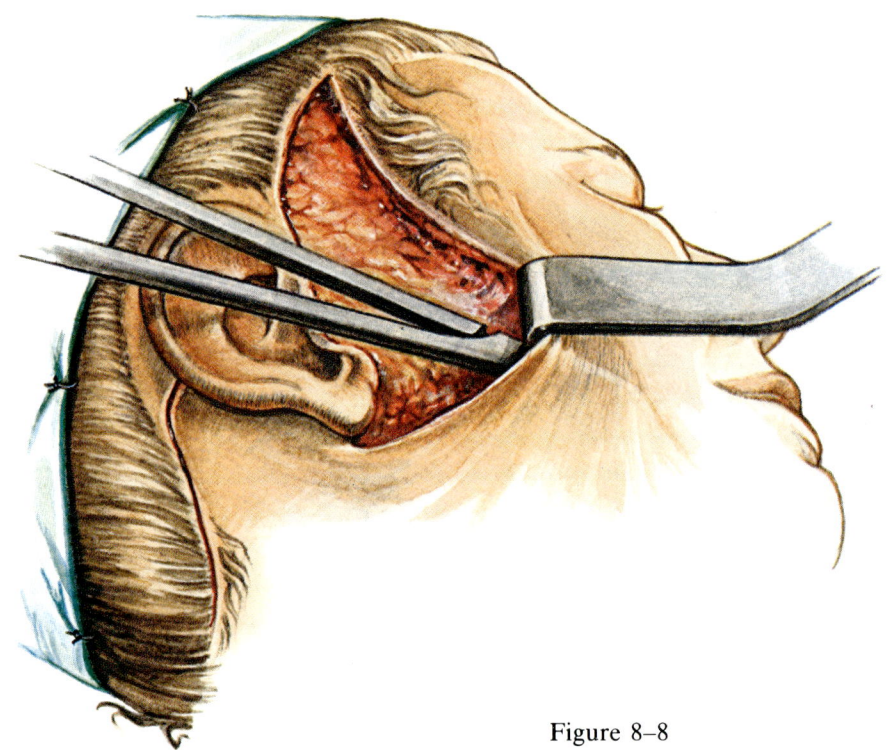

Figure 8–8

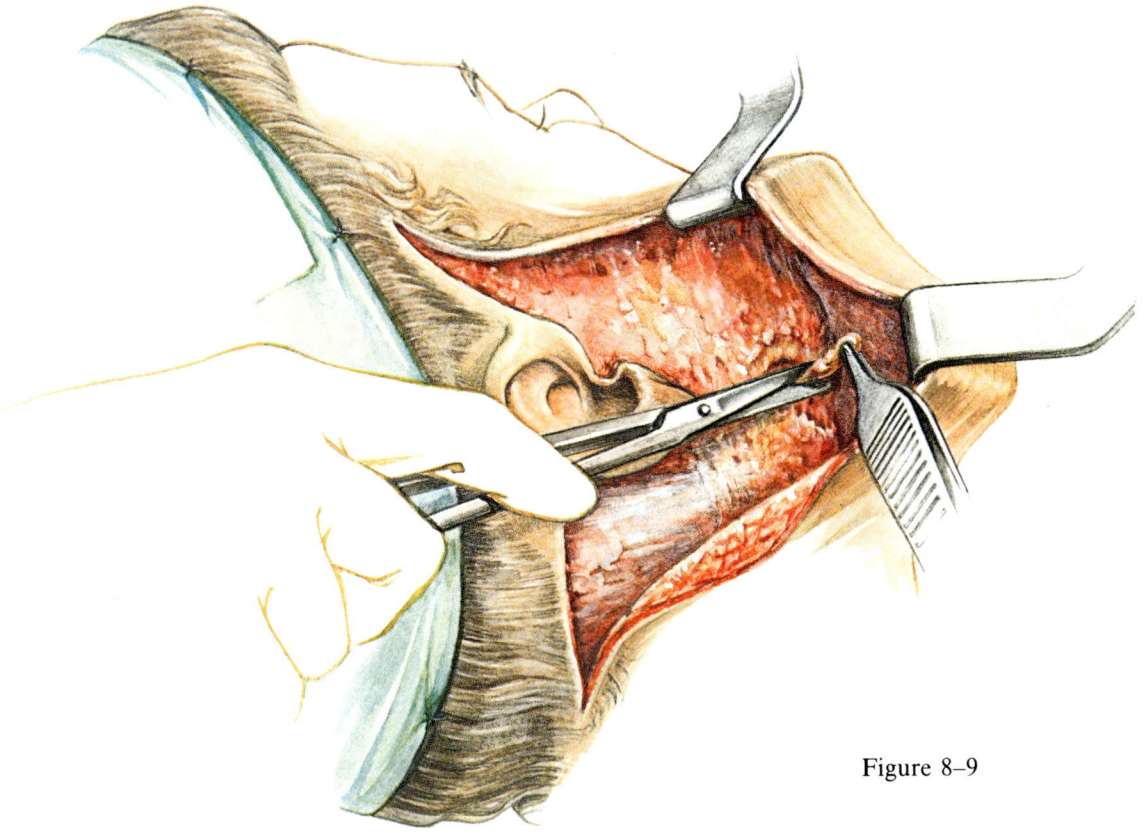

Figure 8–9

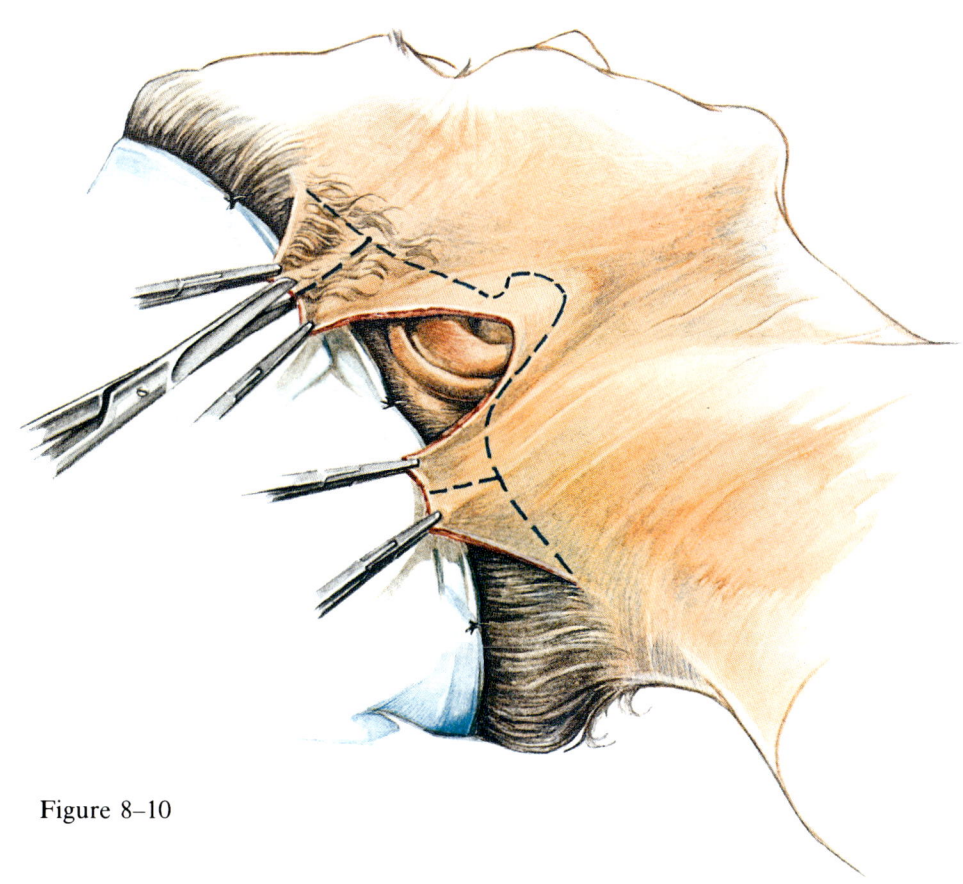

Figure 8–10

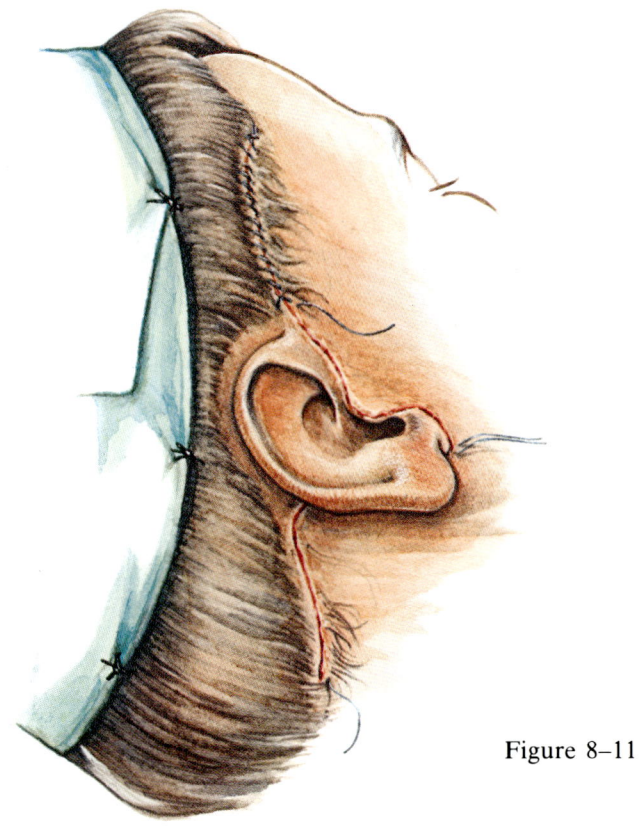

Figure 8–11

the midline of the neck. Most plastic surgeons are of the opinion that sculpting the fat of the neck over the platysma is one of the most important steps of rhytidectomy (Fig. 8–9). This step is aided by a submental incision (see Necklift). After you have completed undermining, place a Kocher clamp on the superior temple flap and another on the edge of the neck flap. Pull the flaps superiorly (Fig. 8–10). Note the effect as flaps are rotated and advanced. Allow the temporal flap to overlap the original line of incision and make a vertical cut in the flap edge until the underlying temporal wound edge is seen. This marks the amount of tissue that you can remove. Hold the temporal flap in place with a single suture of 4–0 nylon. Place tension on the neck Kocher clamp in a posterior and superior direction. Tailor the overlapping skin along the edge as in the temple and hold it in place with a single suture of 4–0 nylon. Locate the earlobe by looking beneath the skin flap and make a vertical incision to allow the earlobe to lie in a natural position without tension. Mark the remaining excess skin with methylene blue and excise it with a No. 15 blade or with scissors. Drains may be inserted beneath the neck flap. You may close the skin edges in whatever manner you choose. I prefer a running suture of 4–0 nylon in the temple skin, a running subcuticular pullout suture of 5–0 prolene in front of the ear, and a running subcuticular pullout suture of 4–0 prolene behind the ear and in the neck (Fig. 8–11). Although it takes longer to place subcuticular pullout sutures, the time consumed is more than made up when the sutures are removed. Another advantage of the continuous subcuticular sutures behind the ear and in the hairline is that no suture mark striae will appear in later postoperative years. Remove the drains and the bulky head-dressing on the first postoperative day and tell the patient to shower and shampoo as soon as her general condition and well-being permit.

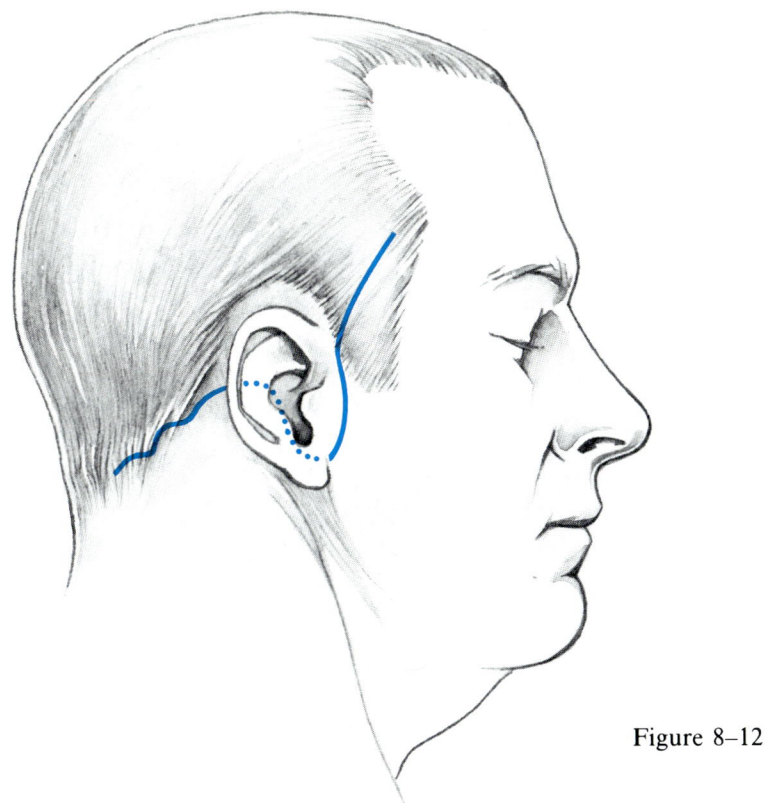

Figure 8–12

Variations

Male Facelifts

More similarities with women exist than differences; nevertheless, these differences are important. Usually, men are larger, their skin thicker, their faces bearded, and their scalp hair more sparse. All of these make dissection in men more difficult and the duration of surgery greater than for women. For these reasons, men are more often operated upon in the hospital under a general anesthetic. The density of hair follicles, richer vascularity, and the greater total area to be undermined make postoperative hematomas more frequent. Hemostasis must, therefore, be complete. The sparse temple hairline and the fine hair behind the neck dictate that the temple incision be made shorter and the neck incision be made along the hairline rather than into the lateral occiput hair. The incision must be in front of the tragus rather than behind to prevent hair from growing into the ears (Fig. 8–12). Also warn the male patient that the neck rhytidectomy will move his hair behind the ear. Although men are more difficult to operate upon because of the technical difficulties outlined, I find that men are more easily pleased with the results.

Temple Incision

Many variations exist for the location and length of the temple incision. A long temple incision allows the face and cheek skin to be drawn superiorward whereas a short incision forces the flap to be pulled more posteriorward. Women with thick hair are excellent candidates for a long incision. The sparse hair of men calls for a shorter incision. A variation of the temple incision is

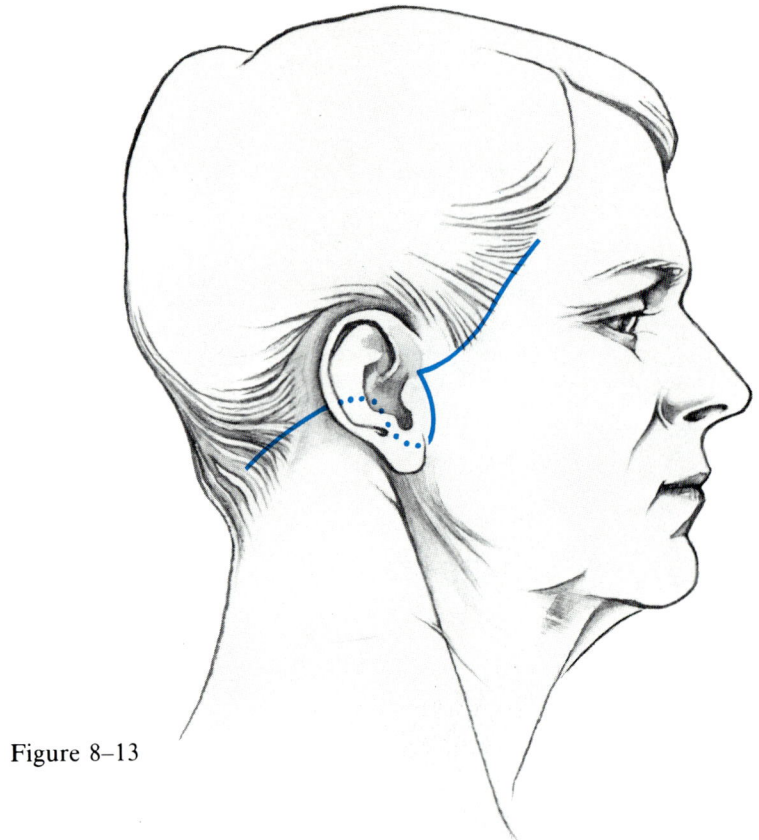

Figure 8–13

to make the cut in front of the hairline (Fig. 8–13). This will allow you to lift the face without changing the hairline. But the final scar is more visible. Give patients adequate information about variations so that they can join you in the decision-making process.

Preauricular Incision

My preference in women is to make an incision behind the tragus. The scar is well hidden and it "breaks-up" the vertical incision in front of the ear. A disadvantage is that skin tension upon the tragus may pull the tragus anteriorward and expose the external auditory meatus. In men, I prefer to make the incision in front of the tragus. The preauricular incision is broken with a "dart" just above the tragus and passes in front to the earlobe. This avoids moving the beard into the external auditory meatus.

Neck Incision

The most common neck incision is to continue the apex of the postauricular incision transversely into the hair of the lateral neck where the hair hides the scar. One disadvantage is that the obtuse angle of the incision makes it act less like a rotation flap. Special measures must be taken to avoid a "step" alteration of the hairline. Secondary facelifts further elevate the lateral hairline of the neck. An alternative incision (which I prefer) is a wavy incision at the hairline of the neck. The more vertical incision produces a true rotation flap and aids in correction of neck laxity. There is no change in the neck hairline and as much skin as needed can be removed. It is especially helpful in the secondary facelift. The disadvantage is that the scar is visible. However, by making the scar in a "sine" wave manner (Connell), and closing the incision with a running subcuticular pullout suture of prolene, the scar is minimal and, in my estimation, a good trade-off. I make this incision as short as possible (4.0 cm) and extend and tailor it as needed.

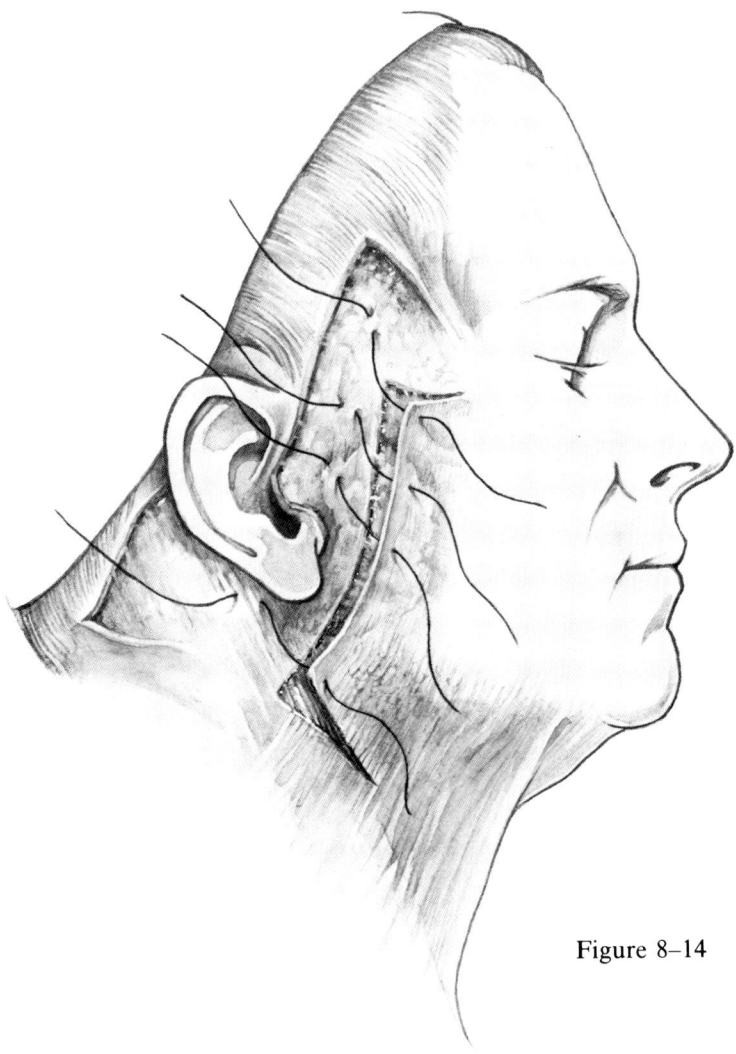

Figure 8–14

Issues

Superficial Muscular Aponeurotic System
The superficial muscular aponeurotic system (SMAS) (Owsley; Skoog) is a continuation of the temporalis fascia which, after it attaches to the zygomatic arch, spreads over the parotid fascia and platysma, and forms the superior sheath of the sternocleidomastoid muscle. Its fibrous attachments to the skin form the basis of SMAS tightening procedures. Skoog and Owsley contend that undermining the SMAS and plicating it produces a simultaneous tightening of the skin.

Locate the zygomatic arch. Draw a methylene blue line from the inferior border of the midzygoma vertically to the angle of the mandible and curve it posteriorly to the anterior border of the sternocleidomastoid muscle and then inferiorward 3.0 cm (Fig. 8–14). Place a small Kocher clamp on the SMAS at the zygomatic extent and another at the angle of the mandible. Tent the SMAS and lightly incise the SMAS between the two Kocher hemostats with a No. 15 blade. Grasp the anterior border of the incised SMAS with an Addison forceps and undermine the SMAS with a fine-pointed Iris scissors for 1.0 cm. Incise and undermine the SMAS and platysma inferior to the angle of the mandible for 3.0 cm. Remember that the mandibular nerve can be inferior to the border of the proximal mandible. At 3 cm below the border of the mandible tunnel beneath the platysma for 4.0 cm, and carefully transect this tunnel with Metzenbaum scissors.

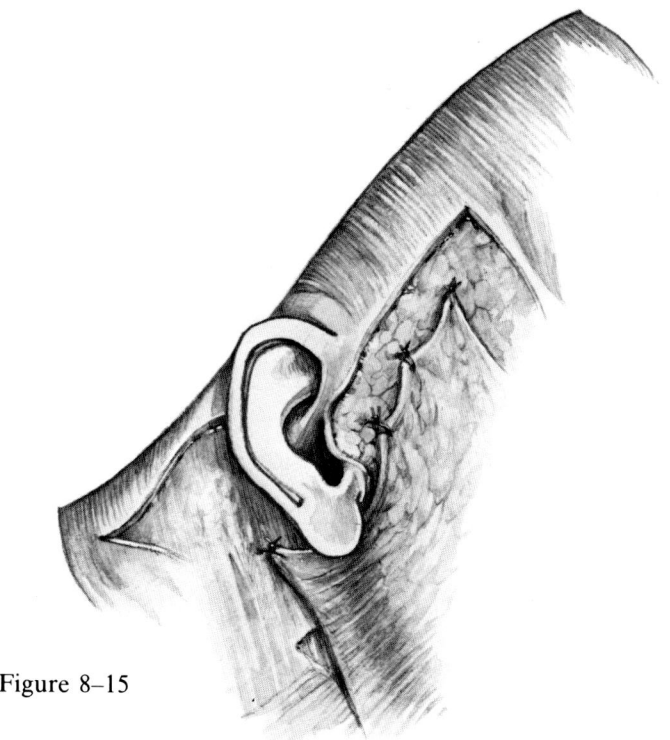

Figure 8–15

The location of the cervical plexus, the great auricular nerve, and the external jugular vein must be reviewed (see Necklift). Place traction upon the free border of the SMAS–platysma flap and observe the transmission to the lower nasolabial fold and upper neck. Rotate the SMAS–platysma flap superiorward and posteriorward and plicate it with interrupted and running sutures of nonabsorbable 5–0 nylon (Fig. 8–15). If the neck does not require platysmal tightening then do only the cheek portion of the SMAS. Conversely, if the surgeon does not believe the cheek needs a two-layer closure, then he is free to do only the platysma tightening.

Improvements achieved by use of the SMAS tightening are largely anecdotal. There is no valid determination of how much improvement results from SMAS tightening. Indeed, Rees, in a series of unilateral SMAS tightening, found remarkably little difference postoperatively.

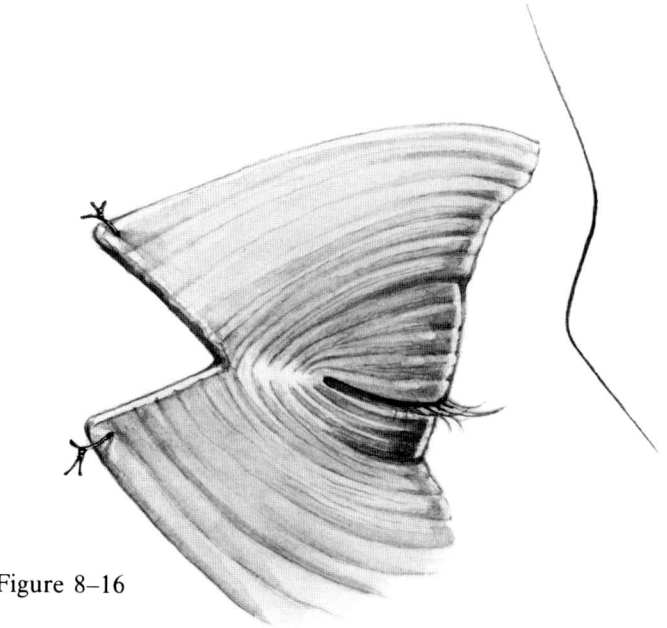

Figure 8–16

Lateral Obicularis Oculi Muscle

The obicularis oculi fibers attach directly to the skin and can be dissected bluntly with a gauze over the index finger. Bleeding may be brisk; pinpoint hemostasis is required. Undermine the obicularis muscle with fine-pointed scissors for several millimeters to form a free edge. Plicate this flap lateralward with several interrupted sutures of 5–0 nylon. Aston transects the lateral obicularis to form two separate flaps. Bring the inferior flap laterally and plicate the superior flap superiorward (Fig. 8–16). This maneuver aids the crow's feet by freeing the skin from the muscle and redirecting the muscle pull. I have experienced two patients with delayed eye blink for several weeks but no permanent palsy.

Additional Reading

Gonzalez-Ulloa M. The history of rhytidectomy. Aesth Plast Surg 4:1–45, 1980. (A comprehensive and very well illustrated review.)

Dingman RO and Graff WC. Surgical anatomy of the mandibular ramus of the facial nerve. Plast Reconstr Surg 29:266, 1962. (An anatomic study worthy of review by all who seek to learn this procedure.)

Connell BF. Eyebrow, face, and necklift for males. Clin Plast Surg 5:15, 1978.

Owsley JQ. SMAS—platysma facelift. Plast Reconstr Surg 71:573–576, 1983. (An update on earlier advocacy of SMAS dissection.)

Rees TD and Aston SJ. Clinical evaluation of submusculo aponeurotic dissection (Skoog) in facelift surgery. Plast Reconstr Surg 60:851, 1977.

Necklift

Jose Guerrerosantos

Background

Bourguet in 1928 first suggested extending the facelift procedure into the upper neck, but he limited himself to cutaneous undermining. Other surgeons who promoted these extended dissections were Crowe in France, Mayer and Swanker in the United States, and Gonzalez-Ulloa in Mexico. Adamson and associates suggested excision of a transverse island of submental skin and fat. Millard described isolated submandibular lipectomy.

In 1971, I reported my experience with plication of the platysma muscle to the sternocleidomastoid fascia. Meanwhile, Rees advocated midline union of the anterior borders of the platysma. Peterson later introduced an "L" incision in the platysma to facilitate its retro displacement. Connell divided the platysma completely in order to form a submandibular sling of laterally rotated platysma.

Today, most plastic surgeons recognize the usefulness of one or more of these maneuvers for improvement of the neck deformity, but opinions vary regarding the extent of dissection necessary in each case.

Indications (Figs. 9-1 and 9-2)

1. Lax skin
2. Flaccid platysma
3. Contracted platysma
4. Hypertrophic platysma
5. Obese neck with submental fat
6. Ptosis of the submandibular gland.

We have defined an anatomic classification of neck deformities at the Jalisco Reconstructive Plastic Surgical Institute in Guadalajara:

Grade I: Mild skin flaccidity or mild fat accumulation without skin flaccidity, or ptosis of submandibular gland.

Grade II: Moderate skin flaccidity or fat accumulation, moderate platysma muscle flaccidity, or submandibular gland ptosis.

Grade IIIA: Fatty necks with abundant fat accumulation, together with skin and platysma flaccidity; perhaps submandibular gland ptosis.

Grade IIIB: Slender neck with severe skin flaccidity; and either platysma flaccidity or hypertrophy, possible submandibular gland ptosis.

Necklift

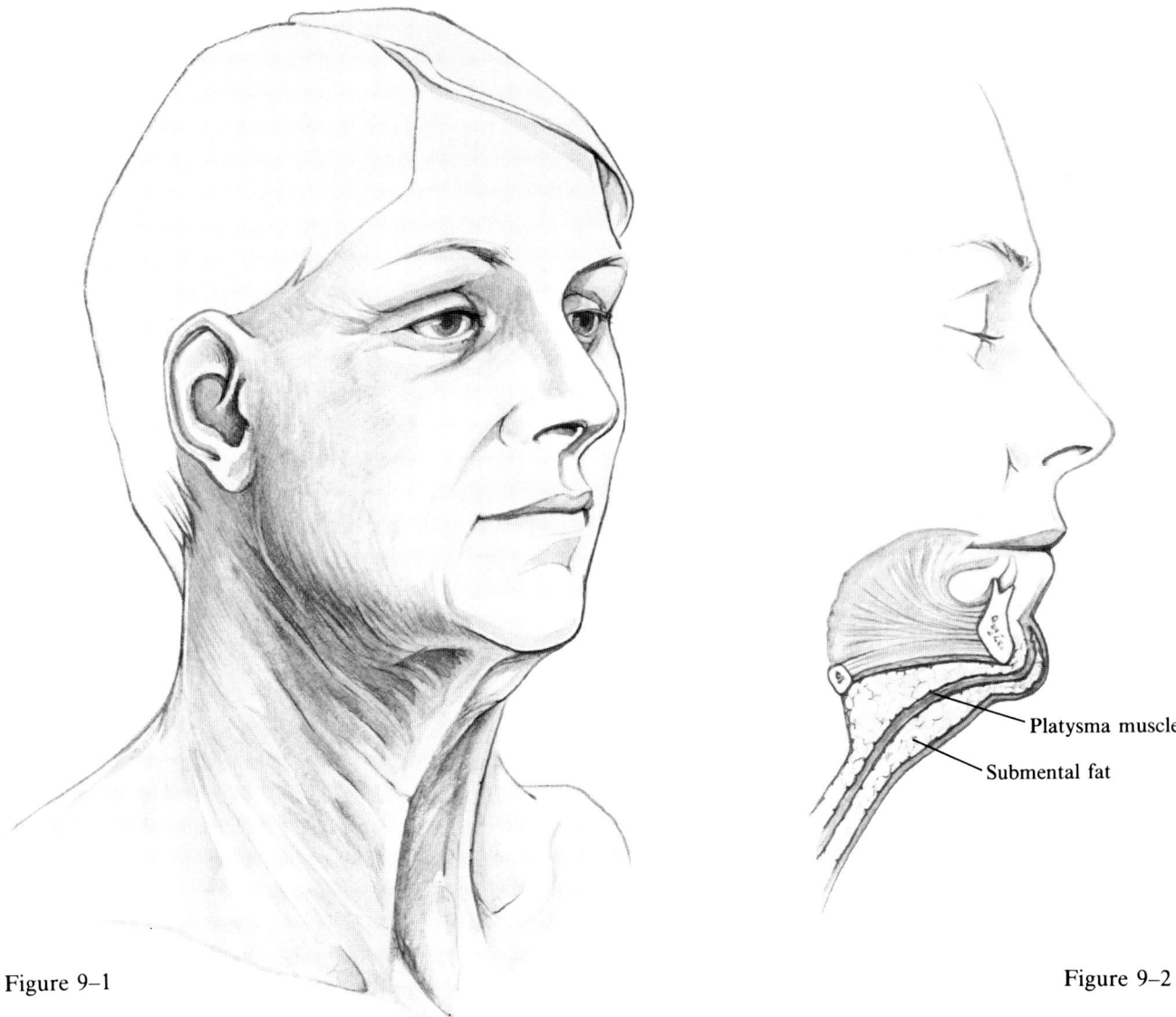

Figure 9-1

Figure 9-2

Contraindications

Absolute

1. Neck skin scarred from burns or irradiation.

Relative

1. Postsurgical scarring of neck
2. Elderly patients with very thin skin
3. Untreated hypertension (increased chance of hematoma)
4. Unwillingness to accept submental scar.

What the Patient Needs to Know Before Surgery

Will Occur

1. Surgical scars (demonstrate their location)
2. Transient skin edema and ecchymosis
3. Transient skin anesthesia
4. Transient emotional depression.

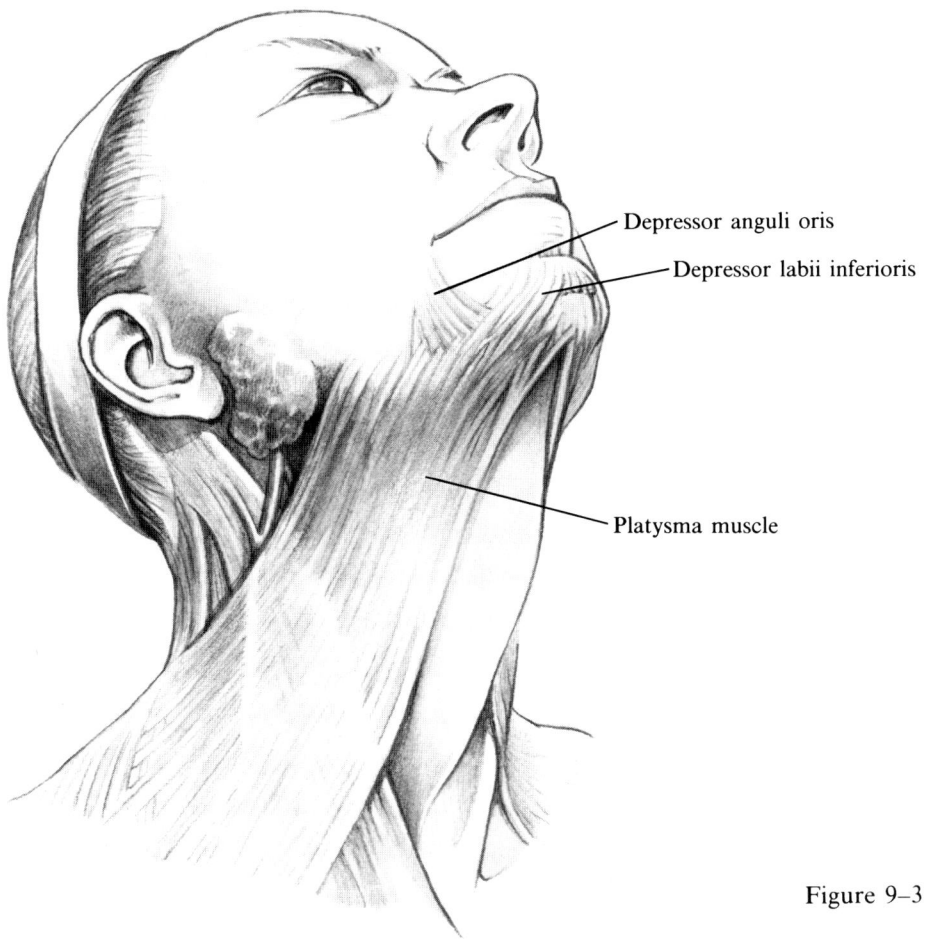

Figure 9-3

Can Occur

1. Hematoma (patient must avoid aspirin or aspirin-containing drugs for 10 days before surgery)
2. Weakness of depressor action of lower lip
3. Change in cervical hairline
4. Postoperative sensation of a "tight neck band."

What the Surgeon Must Know

1. The platysma is a thin, wide, flat muscle that covers most of the anterior and lateral portion of the neck. It lies beneath the skin, attaches to the lower border of the mandible, and interlaces with the depressor anguli oris muscle (Fig. 9-3). It arises from the fibrous connective tissue of the skin near the clavicle and shoulder. Fibers ascend anteriorly in an oblique course toward their insertions. Nerve supply is from the cervical branches of the facial nerve. The action of the platysma is to raise the skin of the neck, as if to relieve the pressure of a tight collar. The platysma also draws the outer part of the lower lip down and back as in an expression of horror.

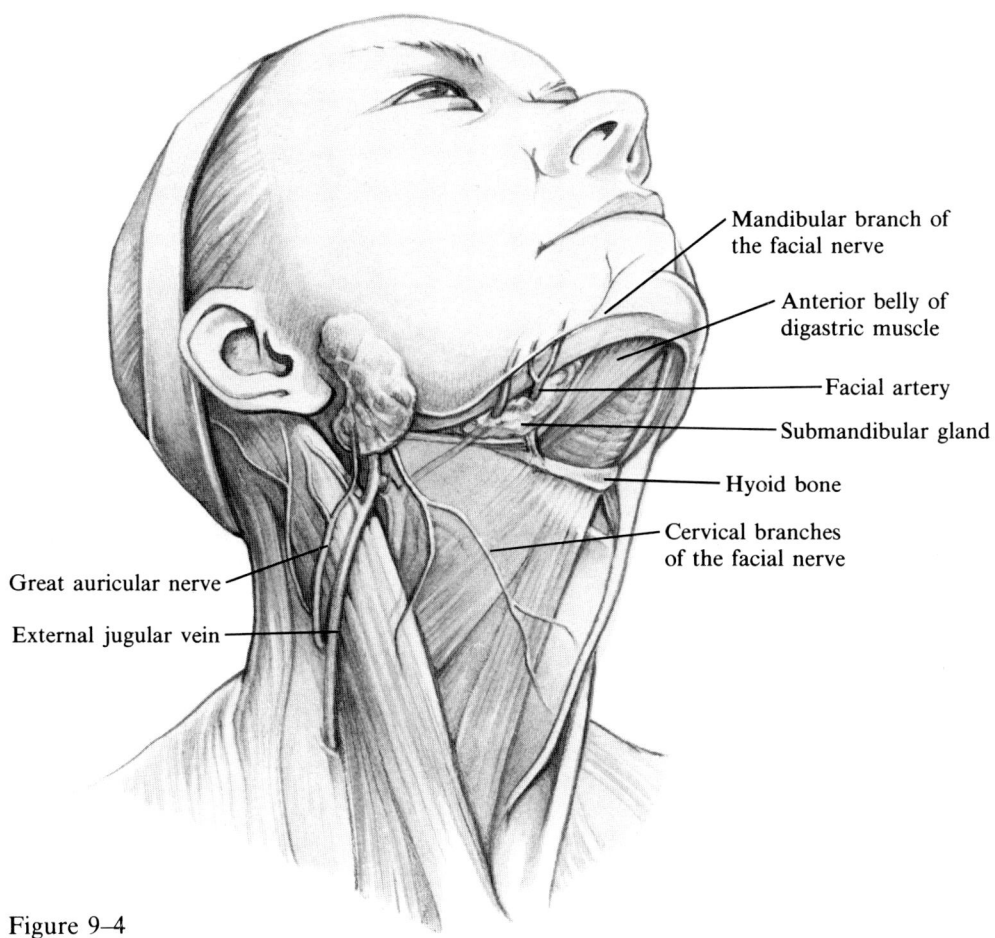

Figure 9-4

2. The depressor anguli oris, or triangular muscle, arises near to the insertion of the platysma and inserts into the angle of the mouth. Its function is to pull the corner of the mouth downward and inward.
3. The depressor labii inferioris begins near the origin of the triangular muscle. It passes upward to insert in the skin of the lower lip and pulls the lower lip downward and laterally.
4. The submandibular gland is situated below the jaw in the anterior part of the submandibular triangle (Fig. 9-4). It weighs 8-10 g. The gland is covered by the skin, platysma, deep cervical fascia, and the body of the mandible. It lies on top of the mylohyoid, hyoglossus, and styloglossus muscles. A portion of the gland passes beneath the posterior border of the mylohyoid muscle. Anterior to the gland is the anterior belly of the digastric muscle; behind it lies the posterior belly of the digastric muscle and the stylomaxillary ligament.
5. The mandibular branch of the facial nerve passes forward and downward, then turns anteriorly to the level of the inferior border of the mandible. It supplies the muscles of the lower lip and chin. According to Dingman and Grabb, in 81% of anatomic specimens, the mandibular branch of the facial nerve passes below the inferior border of the mandible; in the remaining cases it lies above the border of the mandible. Also in a majority of cases the mandibular branch becomes superficial where the facial artery crosses the mandibular ramus.

6. The nerve most frequently injured during the neck portion of a facelift is the great auricular nerve. This nerve takes origin from the anterior branch of the third cervical spinal nerve or from the arcade that this branch forms with the nerve adjacent to it. The nerve surfaces along the posterior border of the sternocleidomastoid muscle about 6–8 cm below the earlobe.
7. The external jugular vein is formed by the junction of the posterior auricular and the occipital veins. It passes superficial to the sternocleidomastoid and then deep, entering the internal jugular vein very low in the neck.

Operative Planning

There are several structural conditions that change with age and affect the neck's appearance:

1. Degree of cutaneous flaccidity
2. Amount and location of accumulated fat in the submental and in the submandibular regions
3. Flaccidity or rigidity of the platysma muscle in both its medial and posterolateral aspects
4. Presence of ptosis or hypertrophy of the submandibular gland.

After careful clinical examination, you must select the technique to be used as follows: (1) Patients without neck skin flaccidity are treated with a classic rhytidoplasty with limited skin undermining. (2) Grade I deformity may be treated with a cervicofacial rhytidoplasty with cervical skin undermining, plication of posterior border of platysma muscle, and perhaps also SMAS plication. Grade II flaccidity requires a submental incision, wide cutaneous undermining, resection of the medial portion of the platysma muscle, lateral plication with the mastoid fascia, and superficial plication of the SMAS on the cheek.

Grade IIIA flaccidity requires a cervical rhytidoplasty with submental incision, wide cutaneous undermining, submental and submandibular fat contouring, medial myectomy of the platysma, and lateral plication of the platysma.

Grade IIIB neck flaccidity is treated with cervicofacial rhytidoplasty, submental incision, wide undermining, resection of the medial bands of the platysma, posterolateral portion, and lateral plication of the platysma and the submandibular gland.

Regional Anesthesia

The neck can be adequately blocked by extending inferiorly the field of infiltration for a facelift. Use of a No. 25 spinal needle limits the number of times the skin must be penetrated.

Operative Technique

Correction of the neck deformity is most often done as an extension of a facelift (Fig. 9–5). The facelift incision facilitates exposure of the platysma muscle. Begin the neck portion of the dissection by undermining of the skin. Remain superficial to the platysma and any accumulated fat pad on top of that muscle.

It is easy to pass deep to the platysma as the neck is entered. This must be avoided! Keep fingers external to the neck skin flap; bimanual palpation/dissection helps avoid entering the deeper plane.

Necklift

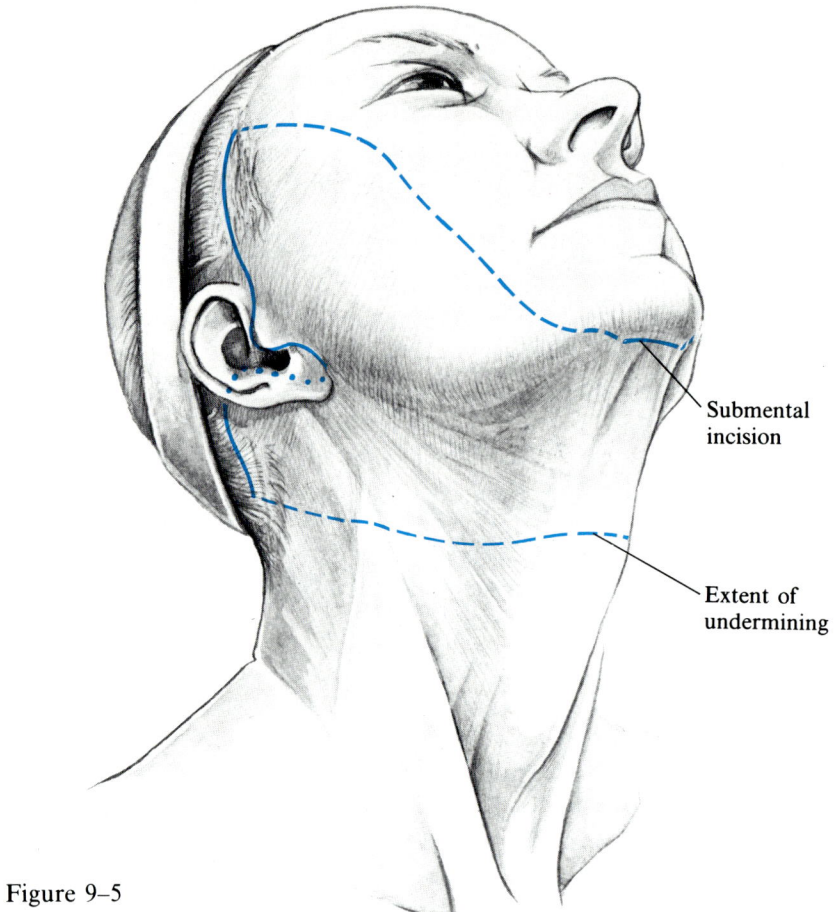

Figure 9–5

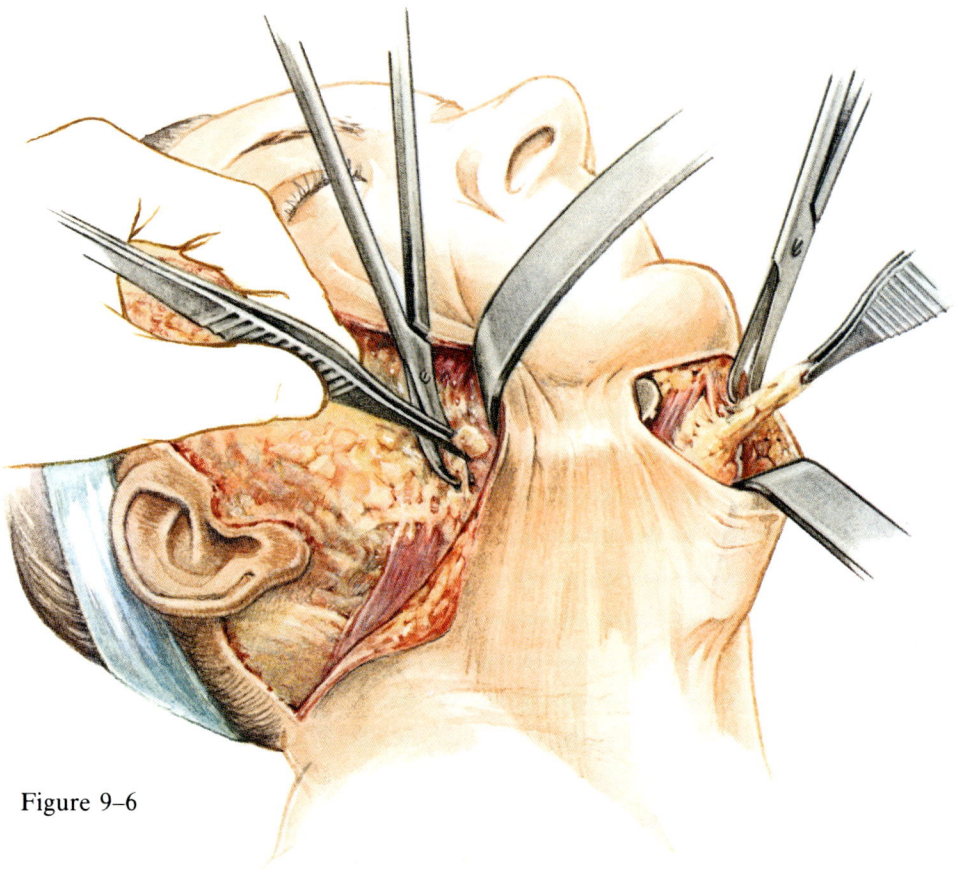

Figure 9–6

Operative Technique

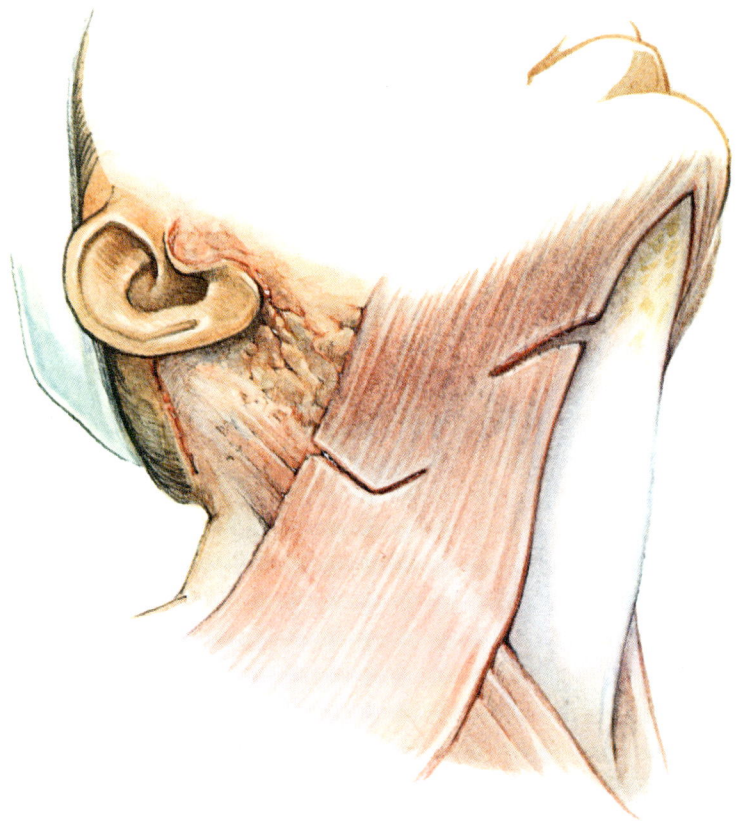

Figure 9–7

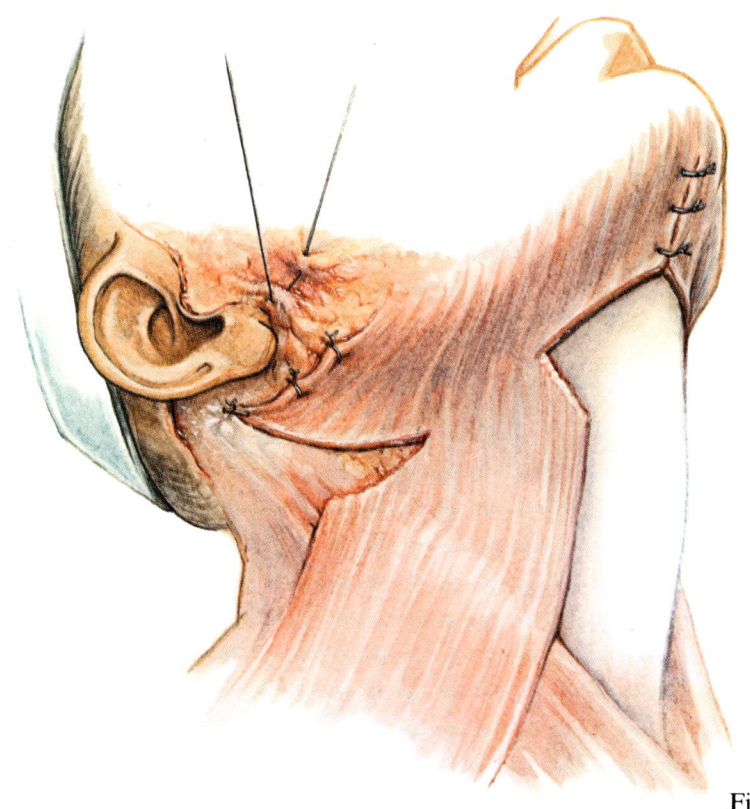

Figure 9–8

81

For minimal neck deformity, fat resection is not necessary. Identify the lateral platysma border in preparation for plication to mastoid fascia. Continue dissection for the entire width of the muscle. Remember that part of the benefit of these procedures is the scar that forms in the dissection plane between muscle and skin. Drain the muscle in a lateral and superior direction. Avoid dissection beneath the platysma, where injury to the mandibular branch of the facial nerve is a potential hazard.

For more severe neck deformities, the lateral exposures on each side must be combined, and joined, with a submental dissection (Fig. 9–6). The midline incision is 3 cm long and placed in a natural groove, or slightly behind the crease. Good results in this region depend on judicious resection of fat. Always leave sufficient fat on the skin flaps to prevent hollows.

Accentuated flaccidity or contraction of the medial platysma border is corrected by medial resection of muscle, or midline plication (Figs. 9–7 and 9–8).

Ptosis of the submandibular gland is corrected by a lateral submandibular–mastoid plication. This lifts the platysma muscle, lifts the submandibular gland, and defines the mandibular margin. Keep sutures well below mandible to avoid injury to mandibular branch of facial nerve.

Variations

Think of the necklift as a medley of techniques, many of them already described, to be applied according to the degree of cervical deformity. Additional variations include interposition z-plasty of medial platysma flap as an alternative to simple plication or resection of the bands (Fig. 9–9).

Issues

I introduced partial division of the platysma low in the neck. Connell has advocated complete platysma transection with lateral rotation and formation of a platysma sling.

Others report a pseudoparalysis of the mandibular branch, which is not the result of nerve dysfunction but rather of excess traction on the depressor labii inferioris.

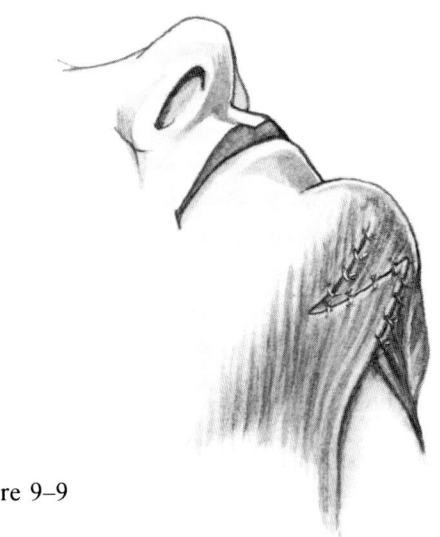

Figure 9–9

At present the trend is away from complete division of the platysma muscle in favor of the multiple plications, medial and lateral, already described and illustrated.

Additional Reading

Gonzalez-Ulloa M. The history of rhytidectomy. Aesth Plast Surg 4:1–45, 1980.

Guerrero-Santos J. The role of the platysma muscle in rhytidoplasty. Clin Plast Surg 5:29, 1978.

Connell BF. Contouring the neck and rhytidectomy by lipectomy and a muscle sling. Plast Reconstr Surg 61:376, 1978.

Vistnes LM and Souther SG. The anatomical basis for common cosmetic anterior neck deformities. Ann Plast Surg 2:381–387, 1979. (This study and the next discuss differing patterns of plastysma anatomic variations in aging neck deformity.)

Cardosa de Castro C. The anatomy of the platysma muscle. Plast Reconstr Surg 66:680–683, 1980.

Millard DR, Garst WP, and Beck RL. Submental and submandibular lipectomy in conjunction with a facelift in the male or female. Plast Reconst Surg 49:385, 1972.

Guerrero-Santos J, Espaillat L, Morales F. Muscular lift in cervical rhytidoplasty. Plast Reconstr Surg 54:127–131, 1974.

Forehead Lift

Matthew Gleason

Background

For many years the forehead was considered a "no-man's land" of facelift surgery. Passot and Miller excised ellipses superior to the hairline. Lexer and Hunt used a prehairline incision. Foman was among the first to undermine the forehead skin.

Mario Gonzalez-Ulloa startled plastic surgeons in 1962 with his innovative facelift incision which neatly circumscribed the entire scalp. He lifted the forehead, cheeks, and neck as a single unit. Even though I visited him and studied his results, I agreed with others who believed his approach too bold. Only recently have we begun to combine forehead lift with facelift. I reported my experience with the temple lift, which alleviates drooping of the lateral eyebrow but did not include the central forehead. In 1974, Jose Vinas in Buenos Aires showed me his version of the coronal forehead lift which forms the basis of this chapter.

Indications

1. Ptosis of lateral eyebrows with or without concomitant laxity of upper eyelids (Fig. 10–1)
2. Congenitally low position of eyebrows
3. Severe glabellar frown lines
4. Horizontal frontal creases
5. Lateral canthal creases (crow's feet)
6. Transverse crease at root of nose.

Contraindications

Absolute

1. No improvement by manual elevation of eyebrow
2. Patient does not want hairline elevated.

Precautions

1. High hairline (especially men) or thin, sparse hair. Make incision anterior to hairline if patient will accept visible scar.
2. Previous blepharoplasty and/or forehead phenol peel

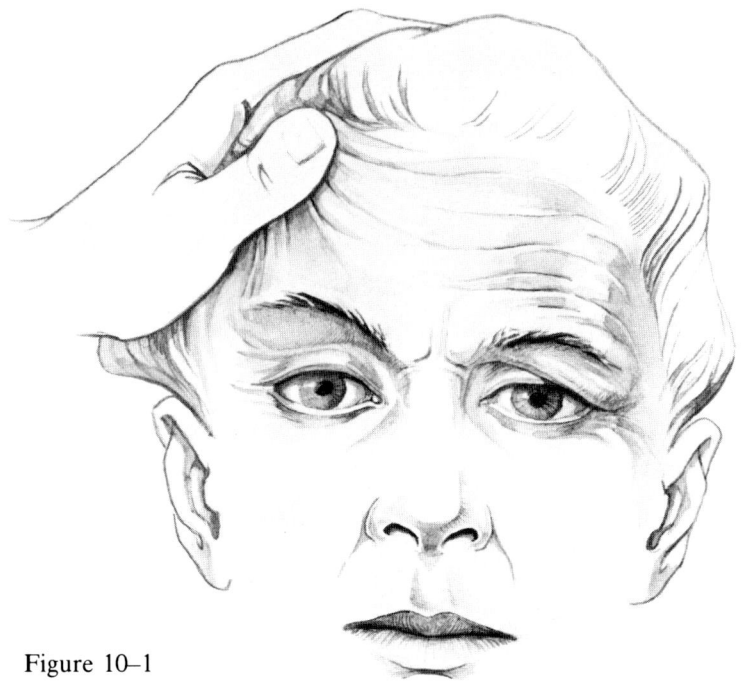

Figure 10-1

3. Thin skin in the elderly
4. Extensive actinic disease of forehead
5. Previous radiation therapy.

What the Patient Needs to Know Before Surgery

Will Occur

1. Elevated forehead hairline
2. Decreased ability to frown (if corrugators are resected)
3. Decreased ability to wrinkle forehead and elevate eyebrows
4. Numbness of scalp posterior to incision (lasts 6–12 months)
5. Hairless coronal scar.

Can Occur

1. Anesthesia of forehead and/or scalp
2. Hair loss (rare)
3. Hematoma
4. Injury to frontal nerve
5. Difficulty closing eyelids (especially following blepharoplasty).

What the Surgeon Must Know

1. The galea is a fibrous sheet arising from the posterior occipital skull; it attaches anteriorly to the supraorbital rim. It fuses laterally with the temporal fascia just above the zygomatic arch. The frontalis muscle originates in the galea anterior to the coronal suture and inserts into the forehead skin and obicularis oculi muscle. The galea is firmly adherent to the scalp but loosely attached to the pericranium (an anatomic fact appreciated by American Indians who were taught scalping by the French and English). The galea is easily elevated from the periosteum of the superior forehead but is adherent to the periosteum of the inferior forehead.

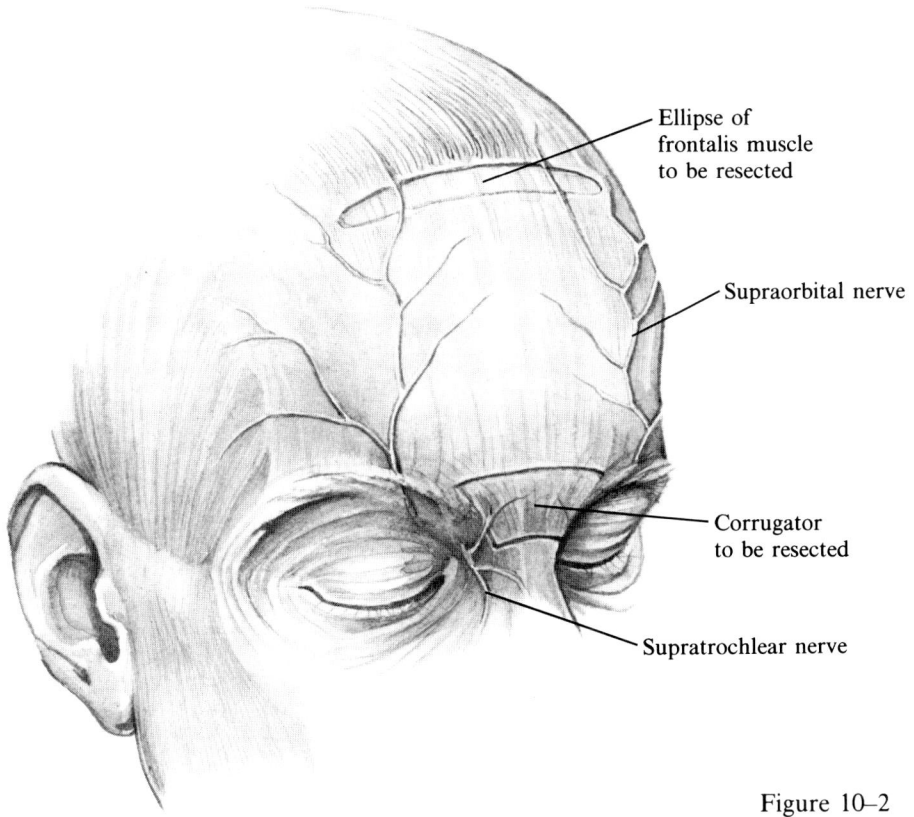

Figure 10–2

2. The frontalis muscle elevates the eyebrows and furrows the forehead; it is innervated by the frontalis branch of the facial nerve.
3. The trigeminal nerve (V) forms three divisions. The ophthalmic division further divides into three branches near the superior orbital fissure. The largest branch, the frontal nerve, enters the orbit beneath the periosteum of the roof halfway to the orbital margin; it divides into a smaller supratrochlear nerve (medial), and a larger supraorbital nerve (lateral) (Fig. 10–2). The supraorbital nerve passes through the supraorbital notch, providing sensation to the upper eyelid and forehead skin as far back as the cranial vertex. This notch is easily palpable on the superior orbital margin at the junction of the medial and middle thirds. The supratrochlear nerve runs toward the medial angle of the orbit and provides sensation to the skin of the medial forehead and superior nasal bridge.
4. The frontalis branch of the facial nerve follows a line from the earlobe to the lateral eyebrow. It passes within the frontalis muscle and is secure if dissection remains deep to the galea. When a forehead lift and a facelift are done at the same time, it is necessary to transect the lateral galea to permit cheek elevation. You risk injury to the frontal nerve if you transect the galea inferior to the eyebrow (Pitanguy and Ramos).
5. The corrugator muscle takes origin in the glabella and nasal bridge. It inserts into the skin beneath the medial half of the eyebrow. It is a wide muscle, and a generous (1 cm) excision of muscle is necessary to lessen a recurrence of the furrow.
6. The procerus muscle arises from the nasal bones and attaches to skin between the eyebrows. Contraction produces a crease at the nasal root.

Forehead Lift

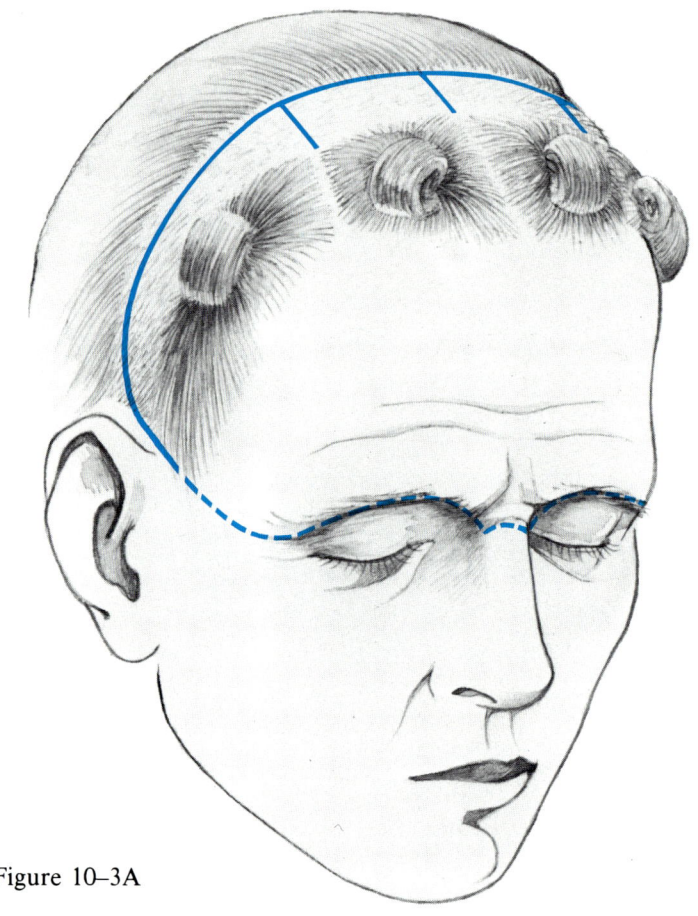

Figure 10–3A

Operative Design

Clip the temple–coronal scalp hair from ear to ear 4.0 cm posterior to the hairline. The shaved zone (2.0 cm wide) is equal to the scalp to be excised. Draw a line with marking dye beginning anterior to the upper helix of one ear; continue across the shaved scalp to a point in front of the opposite ear. This line should hug the posterior edge of the shaved zone (Fig. 10–3A). If the lateral brow needs to be elevated more than the central brow, the lateral advancement flap can become a rotation flap by means of a gull-shaped incision. This allows the forehead flap to be advanced and rotated (Fig. 10–3B). Locate the supraorbital nerve by marking the supraorbital fissure. Outline the vertical frown line to help ensure that the corrugators are generously resected lateral to the frown furrows. Also mark the hairline so if an ellipse of frontal muscle is excised, it will be distal to the hair follicles.

Anesthesia

Identify the supraorbital notch or foramina at the medial third of the superior orbital margin and inject 1.0 cc of 0.5% xylocaine. Create a "furrow" of xylocaine with a No. 25 spinal needle across the forehead at eyebrow level and a second "furrow" within the proposed line of incision of the coronal scalp. Use additional xylocaine as needed.

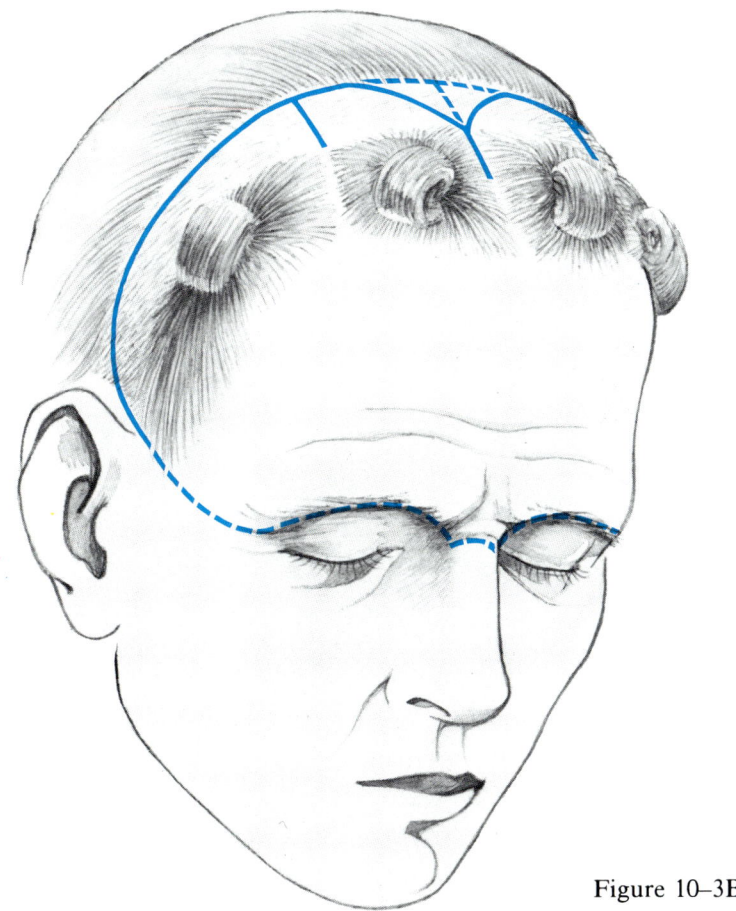

Figure 10–3B

Operative Technique

1. Incise the scalp and galea from ear to ear down to the underlying periosteum. Make three vertical cuts perpendicular to the incision, each 2 cm long (Fig. 10–4). The two lateral incisions are on a line with the lateral eyebrow and the central incision in the midline. These incisions aid eversion of the convex forehead flap and they also measure the amount of scalp to be excised.
2. Lift the scalp and galea with a skin hook and bluntly separate the loose areolar tissue connecting the galea to the periosteum. With a sturdy pair of scissors, undermine laterally to both temples (Fig. 10–5). The galea is more adherent to the periosteum beneath the frontalis. Use a No. 15 blade with the edge held against the periosteum for dissection (Fig. 10–6). Two centimeters superior to the supraorbital foramina, put your middle finger on the skin over the foramina to identify this landmark. Continue dissecting with the No. 15 blade until you see the outline of the supraorbital nerves as they pierce the deep surface of the frontalis muscle.
3. Now use a gauze dissector to mobilize and preserve the supraorbital bundle. Complete dissection of the nerve is unnecessary and dangerous. Detach the galea from the supraorbital rim lateral to the nerve bundle. Unless this is done, the intact galea will prevent the forehead skin from being pulled superiorward. Thumb dissection completes lateral undermining down to the zygomatic arch (Fig. 10–7).

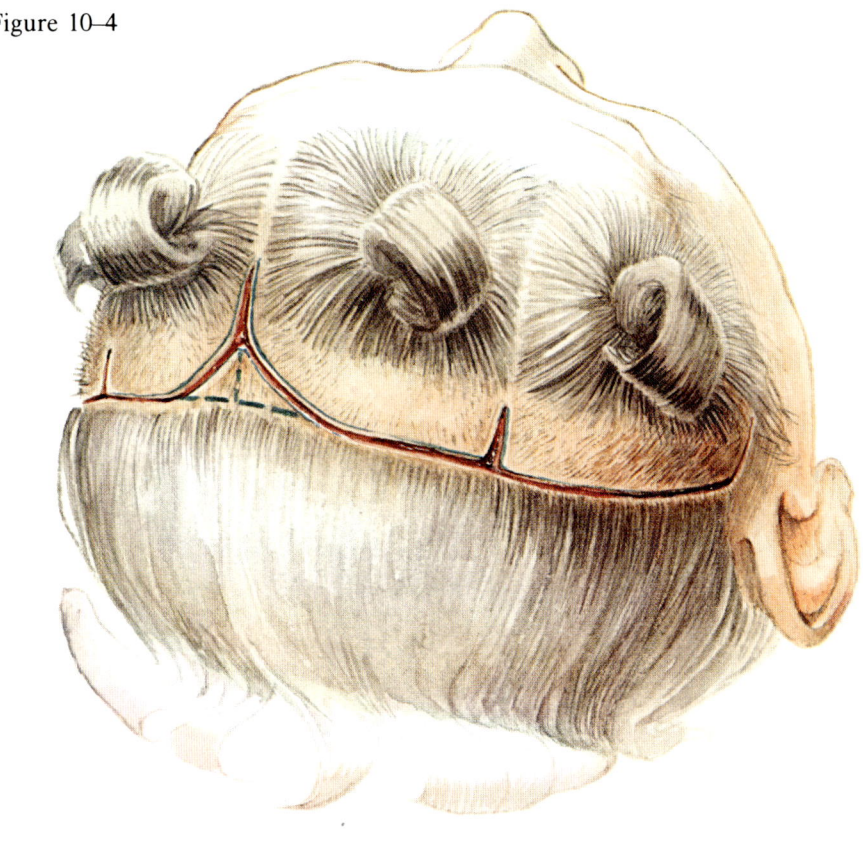

Figure 10–4

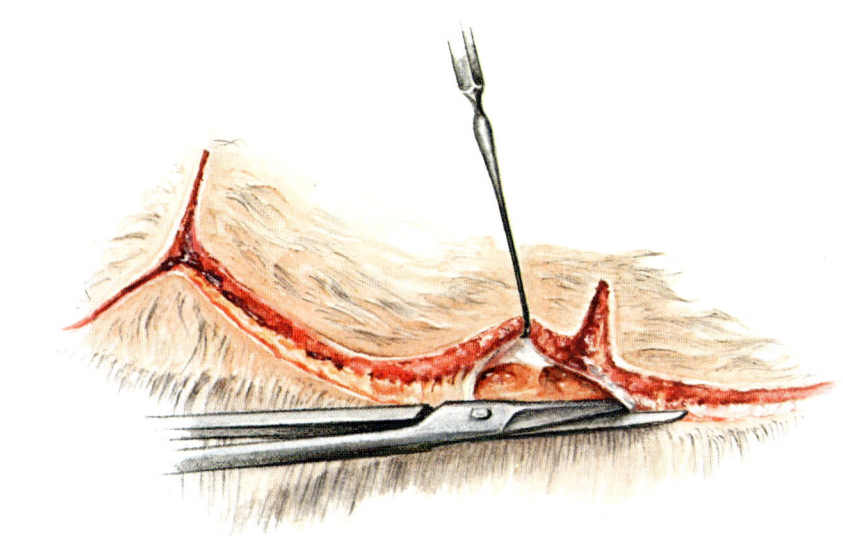

Figure 10–5

Operative Technique

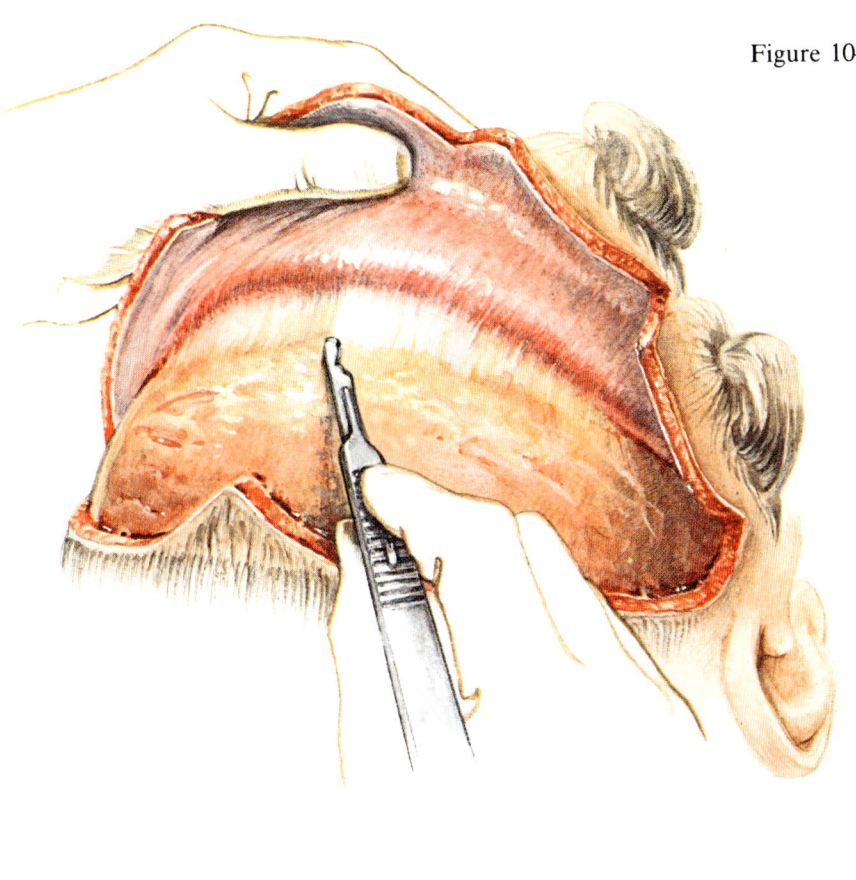

Figure 10–6

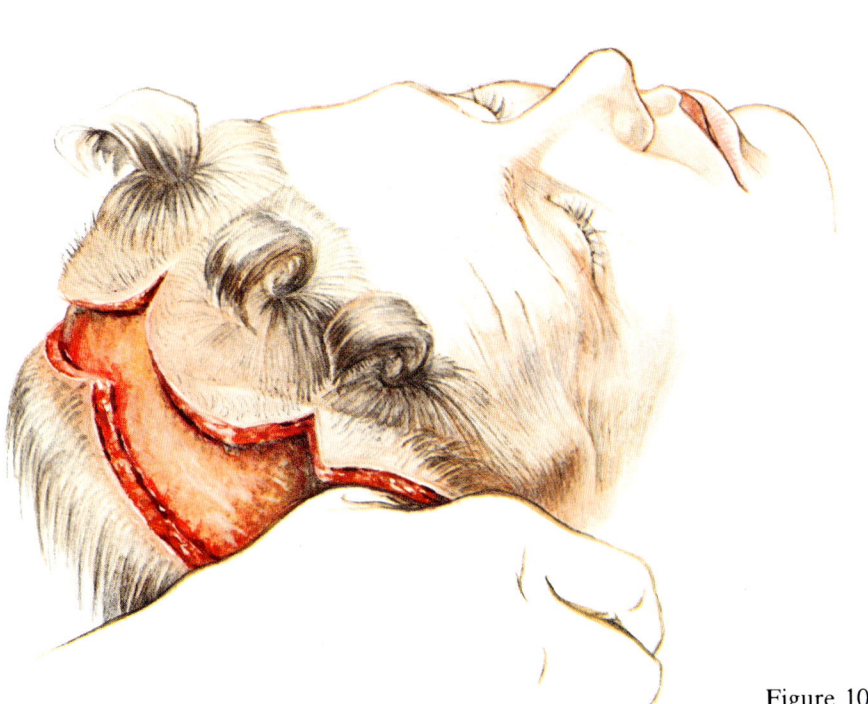

Figure 10–7

Forehead Lift

4. Incise the medial galea attachment from the supraorbital ridge to the bridge of the nose. When the tissues have been sufficiently freed, you can pull the entire forehead superiorward with noticeable elevation of the eyebrow, eyelids, and glabellar areas.

5. Excise a segment of the corrugator and procerus muscles in the following manner. Use a mosquito hemostat to bluntly burrow beneath the corrugator muscle (Fig. 10-8). Start medial to the supraorbital bundle and near the midline. Open the hemostat to create a wide tunnel. Clamp the corrugator and procerus muscles with two hemostats and excise the muscle between them. Cauterize the cut edges of the muscle, and remove the hemostats. If the muscle is removed properly, yellow subcutaneous fat will be seen. The supratrochlear vein is large; avoid it. The wide amount of corrugator muscle removed shows why older methods of relieving frown creases by a direct excision of skin and muscle usually failed.

6. Remove a horizontal ellipse of galea and frontalis muscle from the superior forehead in the following fashion: Insert a needle at the hairline through the skin until the end protrudes through the deep surface. Coat the tip of the needle with marking solution; as it is withdrawn, a dye mark is left on the galea. Make two lateral marks in a similar fashion. Connect the dye dots. This line indicates the level of the frontal hairline. Make a second curving line 1.0 cm inferior to this—completing an ellipse. The ellipse should not extend laterally beyond the supraorbital nerves which you can see as fine, white "threads" superficial to the galea. Lightly incise the galea and frontalis muscle within the ellipse and remove the muscle with curved, pointed scissors until you see yellow subcutaneous fat (Fig. 10-9). Removal of this muscle lessens recurrence of horizontal lines in the superior forehead (Fig. 10-10).

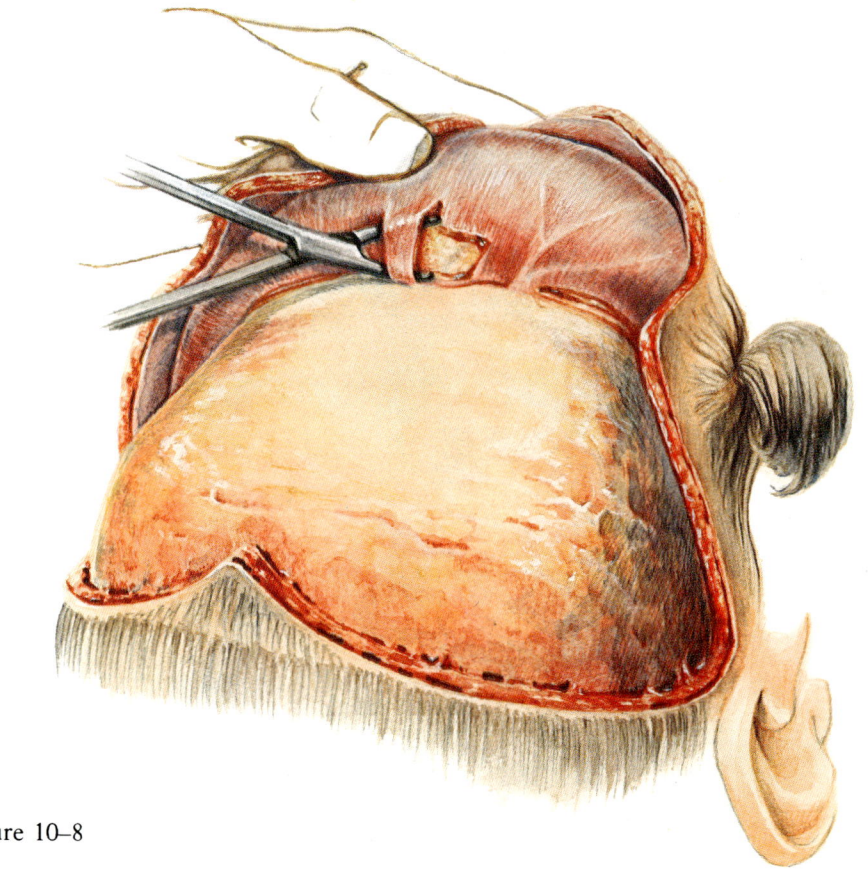

Figure 10-8

Operative Technique

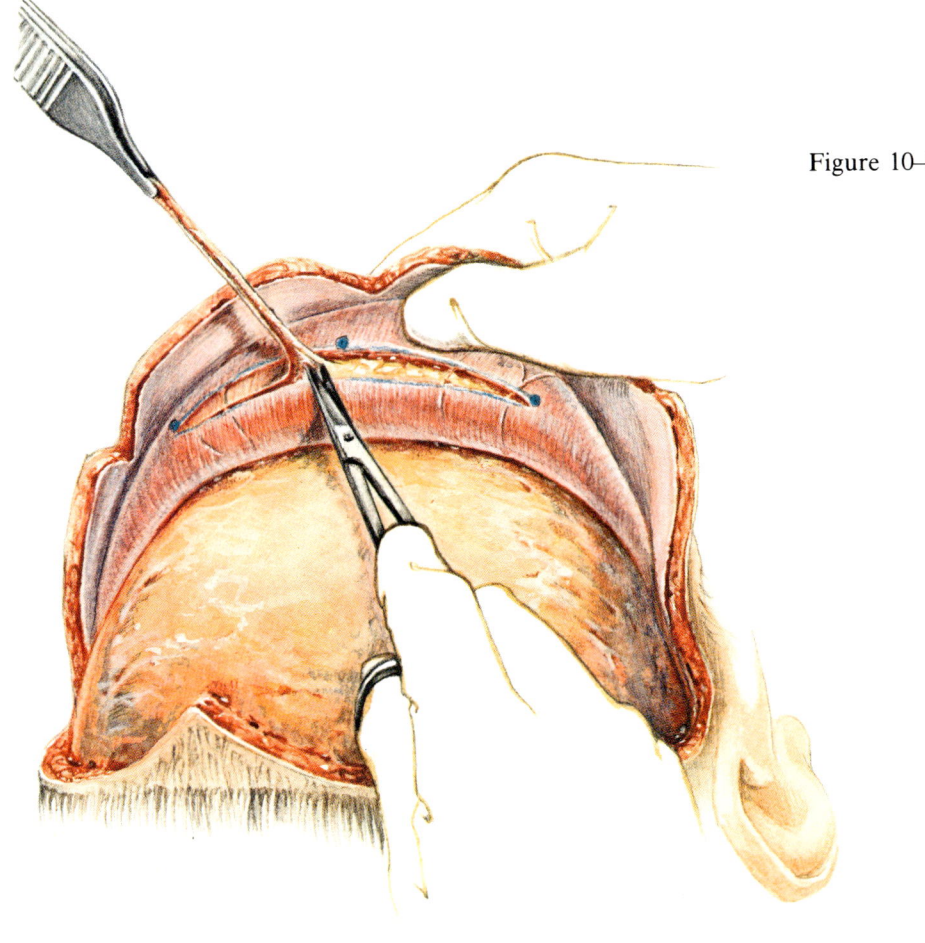

Figure 10-9

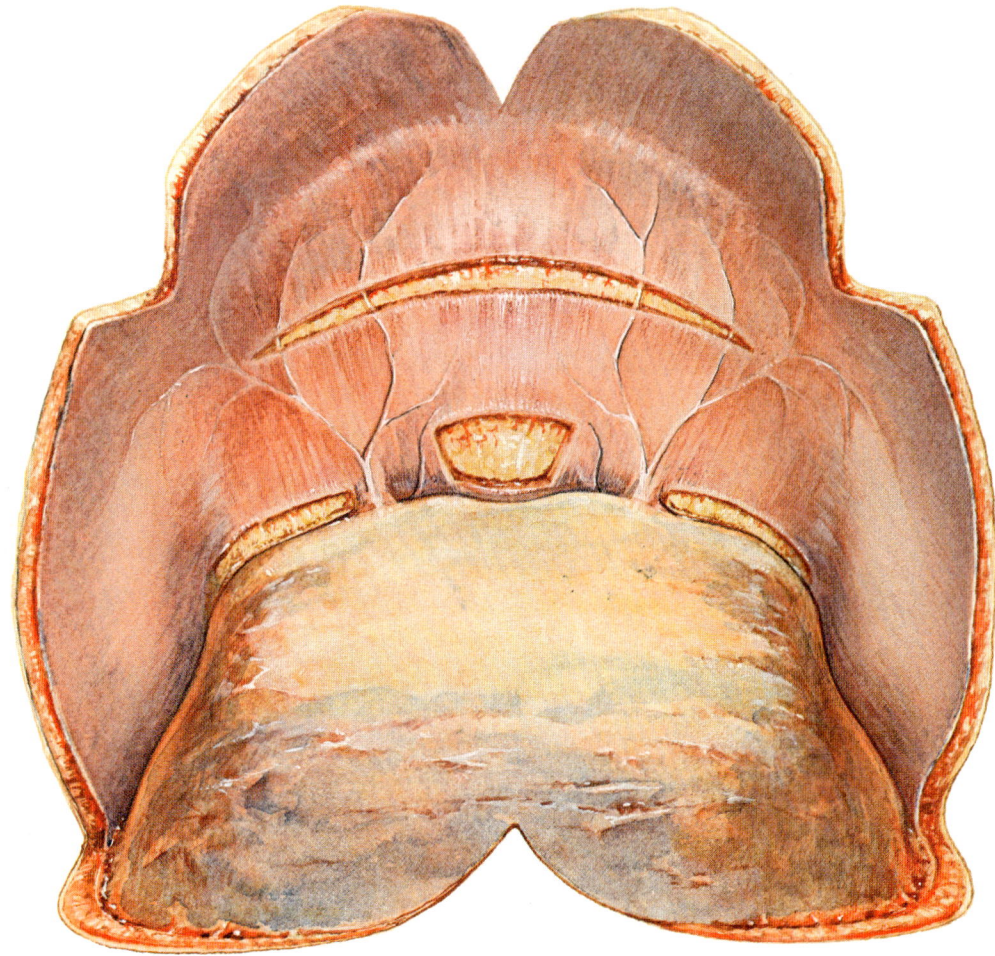

Figure 10-10

93

Figure 10–11

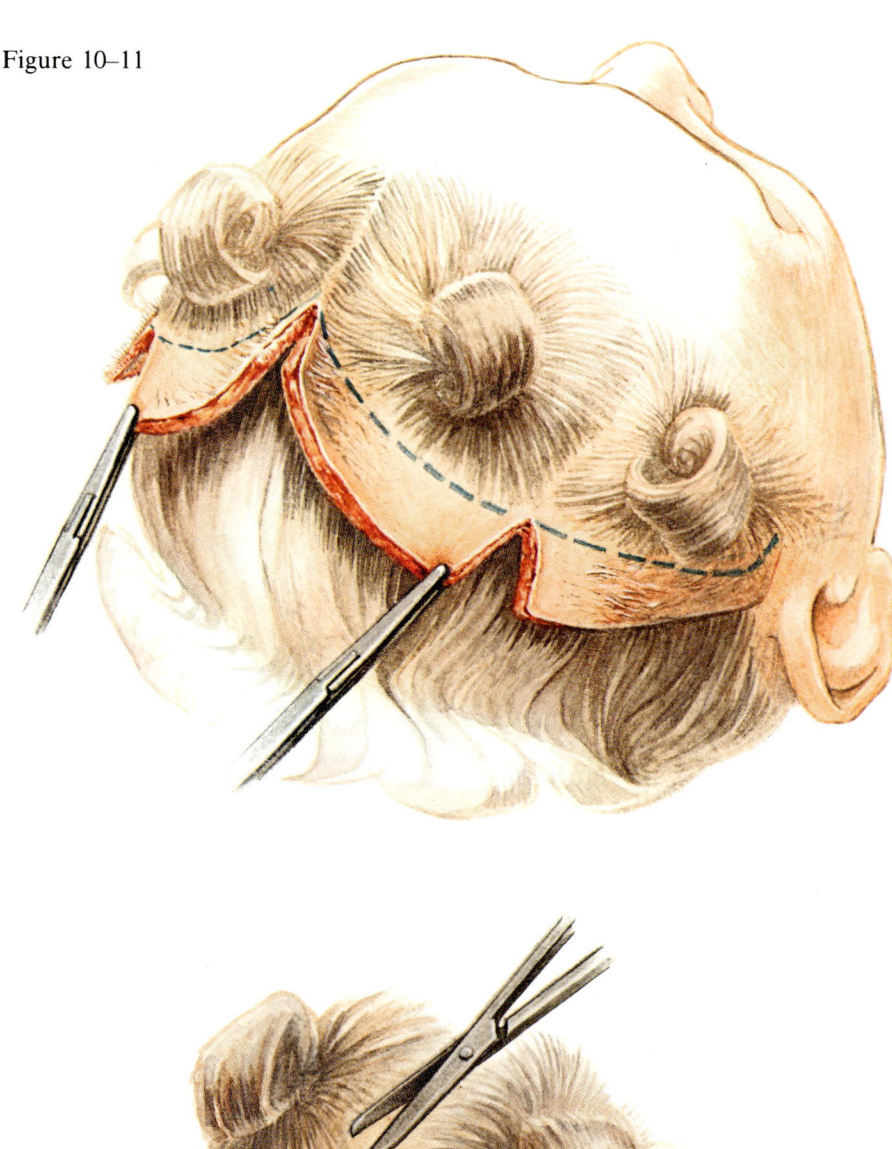

Figure 10–12

7. With Kocher hemostats, pull the forehead scalp flap superiorward, and a 3–0 nylon suture is placed in the three vertical incisions (Fig. 10–11). These sutures pass through the scalp edge and are tied so that the forehead flap overlaps the scalp 2.0 cm. This 2.0 cm elevation will correct the eyebrow ptosis by about 1.0 cm. If there is too much tension, release and reposition the sutures.

8. Cut off the excess scalp (Fig. 10–12). Secure hemostasis, and close the wound with a running suture of 3–0 nylon. Drains are not needed.

9. Place a strip of Adaptic gauze or fine mesh gauze over the suture line. Add several thicknesses of 4″ × 4″ gauze pads and two rolls of Kerlix to complete the head dressing.

Variations

Gull-Winged Coronal Incision

The classic forehead lift is an advancement flap. If you wish to elevate the lateral brow to a greater degree than the central, create two rotation flaps with a V-shaped or gull-winged coronal incision. The point of the apex is close to the central hairline. Thus the entire incision is kept approximately 4.0 cm behind the hairline. If you rotate the flap medialward, and exise the "dogear," the resulting defect can be closed as a "V-Y." Such an incision can be made by drawing an inverted "T" with the long arm of the incision coming very close to the central hairline. The forehead flap is tailored to each case as desired.

Temple Lift

I have largely discarded the temple lift in favor of the more effective forehead lift. However, there are still instances in which I use the temple lift. The temple lift can be done either in conjunction with a rhytidectomy or as an independent procedure. Start the incision in the hair just anterior to the ear and proceed as with a forehead lift to a line above the central eyebrow and stop (Fig. 10–13). Undermine the scalp and galea until you reach the hairline. Next, undermine the skin in front of the ear at the level of a rhytidectomy superficial to the temporal fascia and frontalis nerve to the mid-eyebrow. Join the deep with the superficial planes. Pull the forehead and temple skin

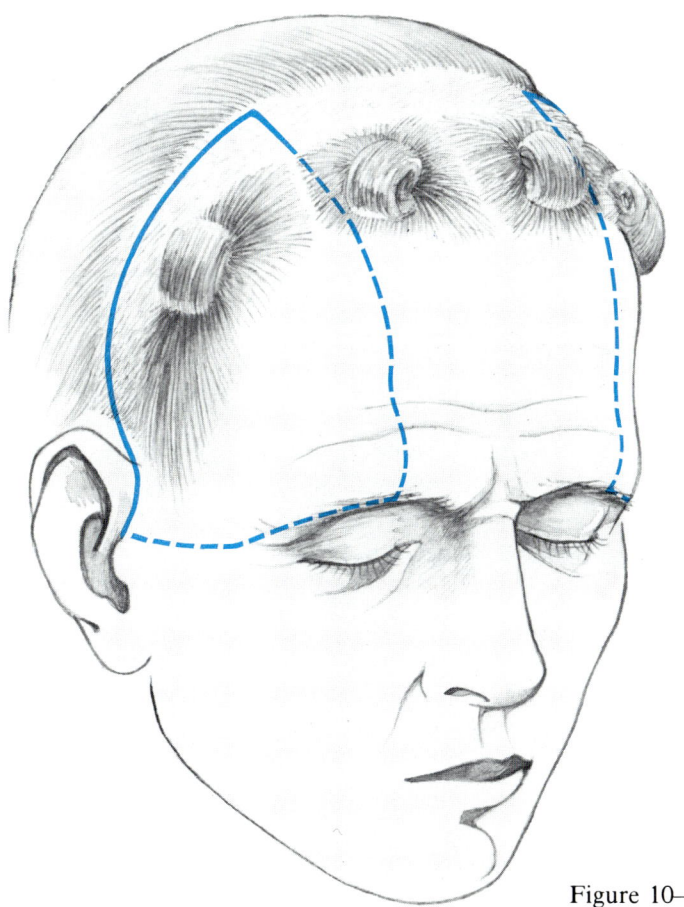

Figure 10–13

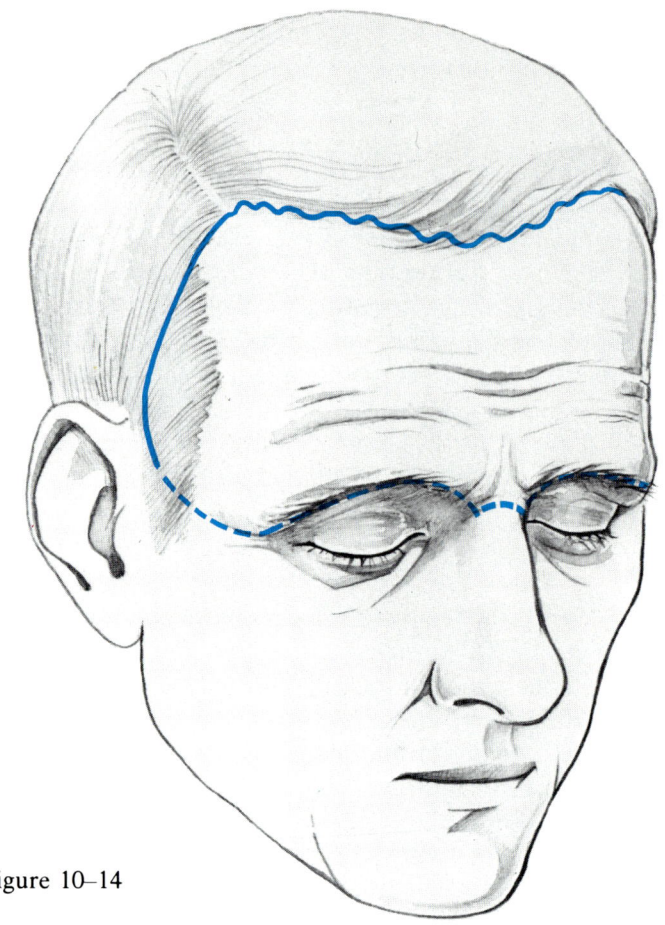

Figure 10–14

superiorward and excise the overlapping scalp. Close the incision in the same manner as a forehead lift. This procedure helps correct the ptosis of the lateral eyebrow and eyelid. It does not aid glabellar lines or transverse forehead furrows.

Forehead Lift in Men
Make an incision anterior to the hairline and in a wavy fashion. The incision in front of the hairline makes it possible to elevate the forehead skin without changing the hairline (Fig. 10–14). I close the incision with a continuous pullout suture of 4–0 prolene to avoid suture marks. I use this incision in women with a high forehead or who have fine, sparse hair. The patient must be aware that the location of the scar may necessitate a change in hairstyle. The scalp directly posterior to the hairline incision will usually be anesthetic from transection of the supraorbital nerves.

Issues

Direct Forehead Skin Excision (Suprabrow Incision)
Only occasionally do I remove an ellipse of skin directly above the eyebrow. This excision does not include the underlying frontalis muscle and I do not undermine the skin. Direct closure of the defect elevates the eyebrow. The thick forehead skin does *not* heal with a fine scar; the scar above the eyebrow is noticeable, so beware.

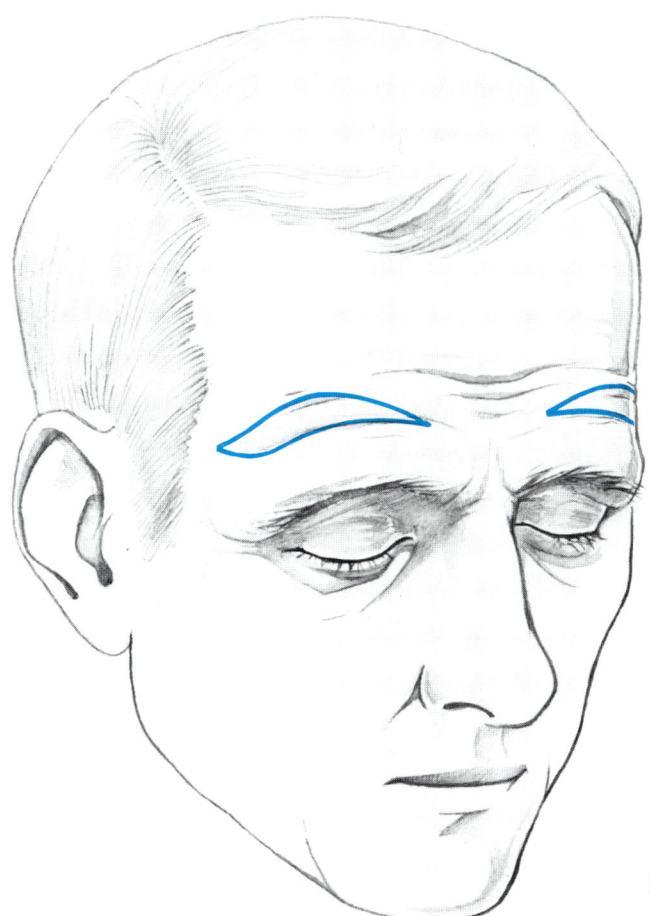

Figure 10–15

In men with deep horizontal forehead furrows, I may excise a large ellipse of forehead skin. Keep the inferior incision in a furrow closest to the eyebrow (Fig. 10–15). Only rarely does a forehead furrow run in a continuous line from one side of the forehead to the other. More often it is broken, and one side is at a different level than the other. Take advantage of this asymmetry because two scars at slightly different levels are not as noticeable as a single scar running across the entire forehead. Do not undermine. Stay superficial to the frontalis muscle; avoid the frontalis nerve and the supraorbital nerve. The amount of skin to be removed is commonly underestimated. Excise a generous amount; then with the patient in a sitting position, use a suture to close the incision and judge the amount of improvement. Excise additional skin as needed.

Direct Frown Excision
It is impossible to correct glabellar frown lines by direct excision. Forehead skin is thick and the surgical scar is very similar to the glabellar frown removed. The amount of corrugator that you can remove through this limited approach is minimal. Experience with the forehead lift demonstrates that the corrugator muscle arising from the glabellar area has a wide insertion into the medial skin of the forehead. A strip of corrugator at least a centimeter wide must be removed to inhibit early return of the corrugator action. A direct approach removes only a small segment of the corrugator, and the corrugator action is not sufficiently interrupted.

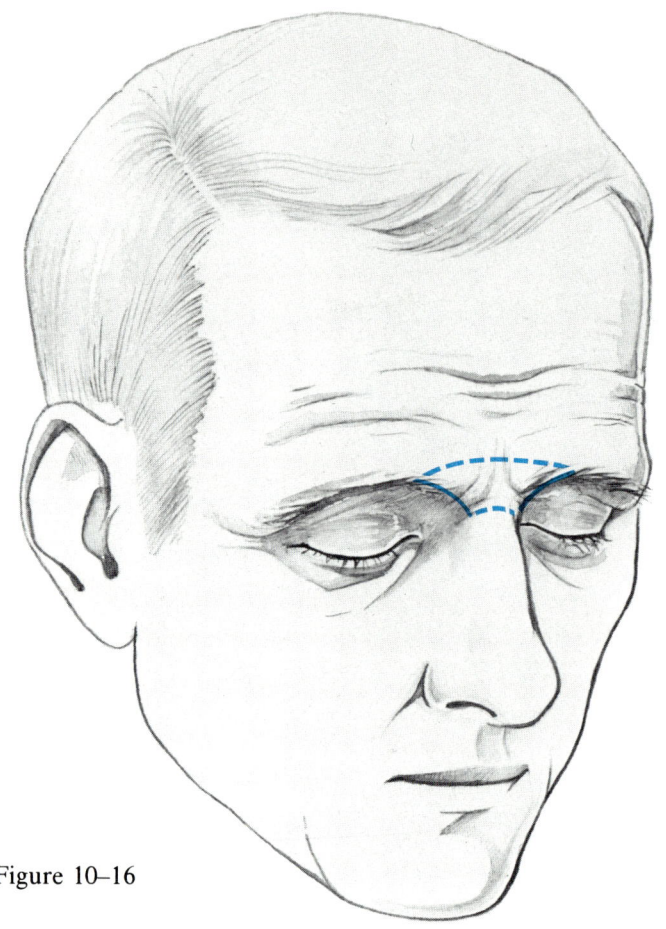

Figure 10-16

One alternative is a horizontal incision made directly in the medial eyebrow (Fig. 10–16). Undermine the skin as a tunnel to join the two incisions. Use a small Joseph rhinoplasty elevator to expose the corrugator and procerus muscles. Two mosquito hemostats are introduced through the incisions. The inferior hemostat is placed close to the insertion near the nasal bridge. The more superior hemostat is clamped 1.0 cm above. The muscle is transected and cauterized. The excised muscle is thin and its absence will not result in a depression. Do not attempt to excise the vertical frown line.

Additional Reading

Gonzales Ulloa M. The history of rhytidectomy. Aesth Plast Surg 4:1–45, 1980.

Pitanguy I and Ramos AS. The frontal branch of the facial nerve: Importance of its variations in facelifting. Plast Reconstr Surg 38:452–456, 1966.

Vinas J, Caviglia C, Cortinos J. Forehead rhytidoplasty and brow lifting. Plast Reconstr Surg 57:445, 1976.

Gleason MC. Brow lifting through a temporal scalp approach. Plast Reconstr Surg 52:141, 1973.

Rhinoplasty

Leonard W. Glass and Thomas Donovan

The final surgical procedure to be discussed is corrective rhinoplasty, not because of the topic's relative unimportance, but because of its complexity and challenge. Procedures discussed previously will be mastered more easily, perhaps within the residency training interval. Rhinoplasty remains a challenge well into a plastic surgeon's career. It is essentially a blind procedure, perhaps least predictable of all the tissue manipulations attempted by a reconstructive surgeon.

This discussion is by no means complete. It is a beginning point, referenced for additional reading. Our residents are asked to begin their study of rhinoplasty very early, but to attempt their "first noses" under close supervision after other aesthetic procedures are learned. They leave training with confidence in their overall approach to aesthetic surgery, a satisfactory experience with rhinoplasty, yet with lingering doubts and an unfinished learning agenda for corrective nasal surgery.

Background

Corrective rhinoplasty can be considered a 19th century innovation. Diffenbach used external incisions to alter nasal contour. But modern rhinoplasty technique begins with Joseph, whose Berlin clinic made him and nasal surgery famous. His surgical approach to the deformed nasal skeleton was through intranasal incisions, a very significant advance! His techniques were introduced into America by Aufricht and by Safian. Many others have since contributed to a more sophisticated understanding of the complex relationship between nasal function and nasal aesthetics, most notably Sheen.

Indications (Fig. 11-1)

1. Prominent nasal dorsum
2. Excessive dorsal length
3. Excessive dorsal width
4. Dorsal asymmetry (deviated nose)
5. Excess or inadequate tip projection
6. Acute nasolabial angle (hanging tip)
7. Obtuse nasolabial angle (tethered upper lip)
8. Bulbous tip
9. Abnormal columella–ala relationship
10. Airway obstruction.

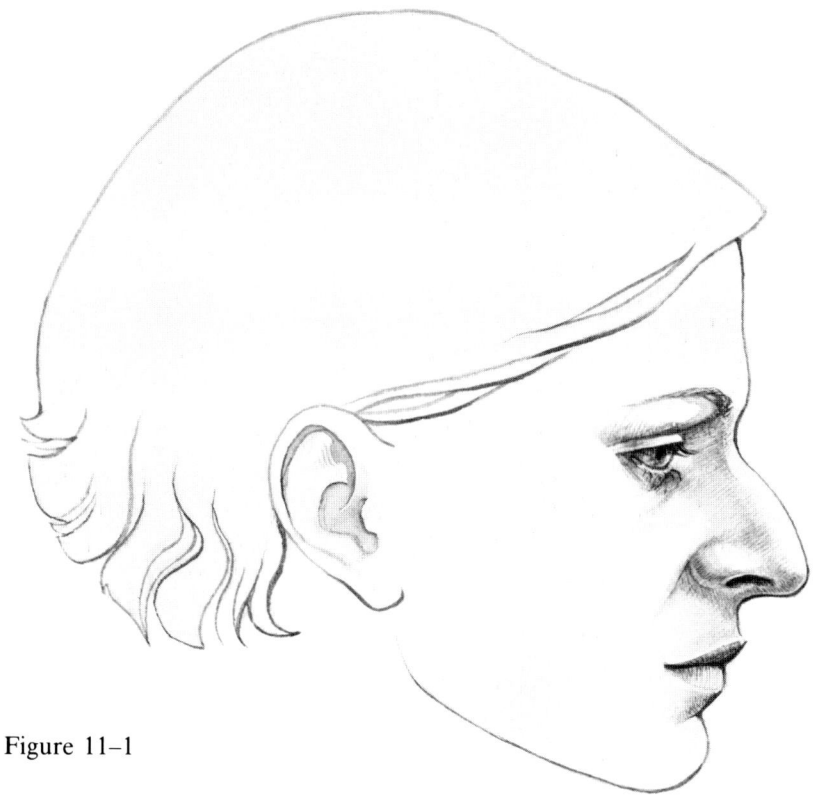

Figure 11-1

Potential Contraindications

1. Unreasonable patient expectation
2. Thickened (sebaceous) nasal skin
3. Thin, sun damaged, or X-ray damaged nasal skin
4. Malignancy of nasal skin
5. Short nasal bones or narrow cartilaginous vault
6. Straight dorsum (do not overresect)
7. Inadequate or marginal tip projection
8. High septal deviation
9. Prognathism (nasal reduction worsens facial balance)
10. Prior patient dissatisfaction.

What the Patient Needs to Know Before Surgery

Will Occur

1. Nasal and periorbital bruising for 2-3 weeks
2. Nasal obstruction and drainage for 3-6 weeks
3. Nasal edema for 6-12 weeks
4. Nasal pack for 3-5 days
5. Nasal splint for 1 week
6. No strenuous exercise for 1 month.

Can Occur

1. Nasal skeletal irregularity
2. Asymmetry

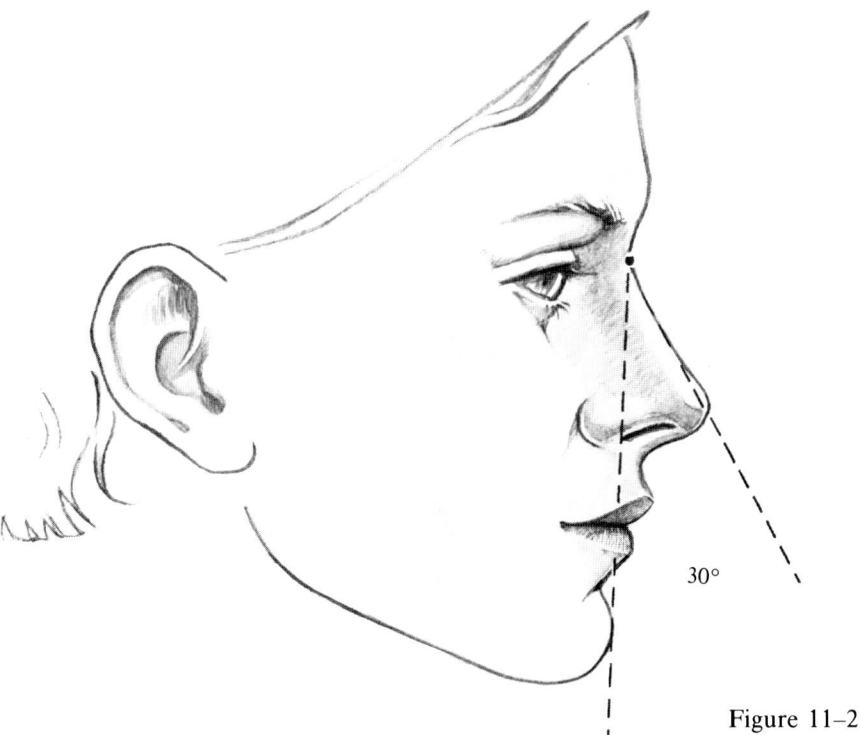

Figure 11-2

3. Dysesthesia, anesthesia of nasal tip
4. Diminished nasal airway
5. Dropped tip or "polly break deformity"
6. Excessively narrow nose
7. Other occurrences, less common, include: lacrimal obstruction, eyelid discoloration, pinched tip, septal perforation, epistaxis, smile change, saddle deformity, skin necrosis.

What the Surgeon Must Know

1. Aesthetics: In profile, the idealized nose has a straight dorsum forming a 30–35° angle with the facial perpendicular (Fig. 11–2). The dorsum represents an uninterrupted continuation of the supraorbital line. The tip is the highest point of the profile, rising slightly above the dorsum. The nasolabial angle is 10–15° in males, 15–25° in females. The facial perpendicular from nasion to columellar base also crosses the tip of the chin. The columella projects 3–5 mm below the alar rims. In frontal view, the supraorbital line flows uninterrupted along the bridge to the nasal tip (Fig. 11–3). Domes of the lower lateral cartilages form two equilateral triangles with the columellar lobular junction and the point where the tip rises above the dorsum. Nostrils are elliptical and oriented as a triangle from base to tip (Fig. 11–4).
2. Structural anatomy: A thorough understanding of nasal anatomy is mandatory for development of rhinoplasty skill, and will not be duplicated in this discussion. Readers are directed to scholarly renderings on this subject in monographs by Rees and Sheen.

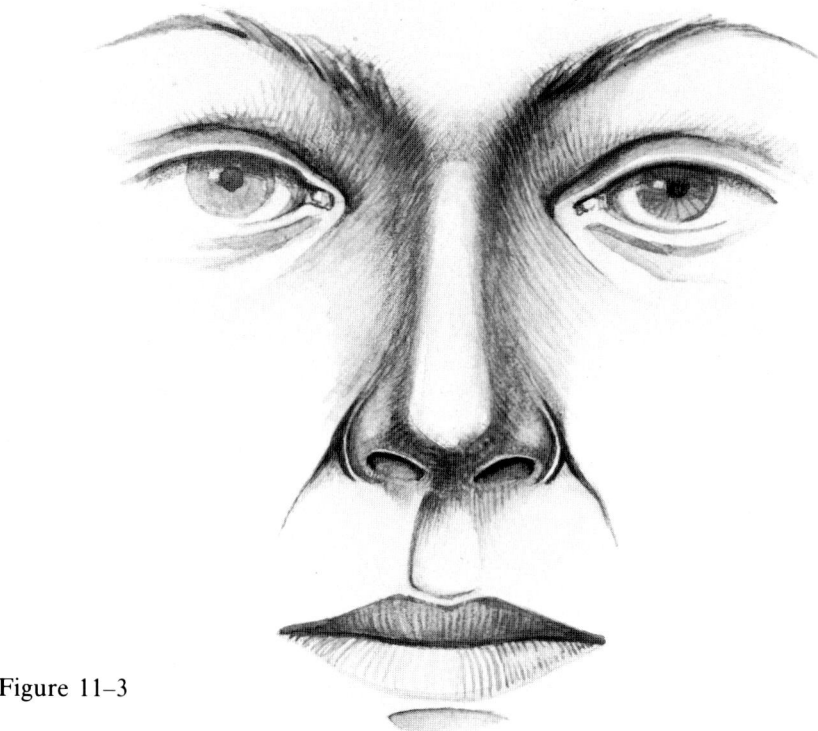

Figure 11-3

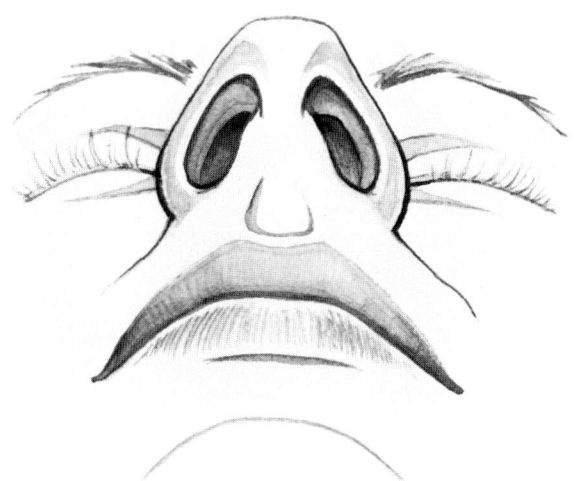

Figure 11-4

Operative Planning

Rhinoplasty is *not* a single operation. It is like a medley of several maneuvers, custom-assembled to meet specific patient and surgeon goals. Operative design therefore proceeds as careful preoperative nasal evaluation takes place.

Preoperative Evaluation

1. Profile: Check dorsal line (questionable hump, questionable saddle), dorsum–tip relationship, nasolabial angle, tip outline, columella–ala relationship, nose–chin relationship.

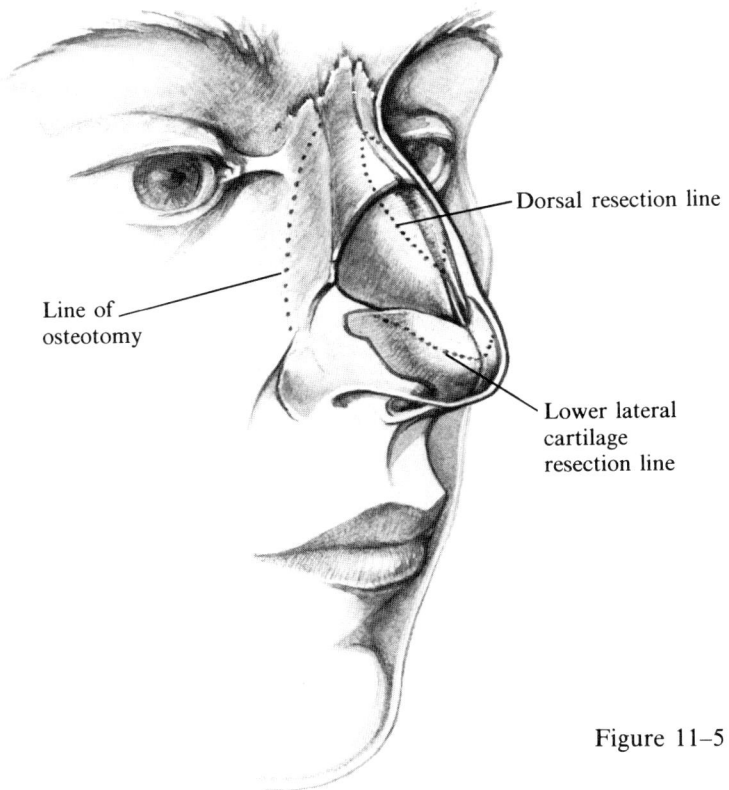

Figure 11-5

2. Frontal: Check for bony deviation, widened bridge, tip configuration, nature and thickness of overlying skin.
3. Basal: Check nostril size and shape, columellar then note bridge again for symmetry and/or asymmetry.
4. Internal: Determine septal position; check for turbinate hypertrophy, valve, function, stenosis, perforation, synechiae (mucosal adhesions).

Preoperative Marking
With experience, many rhinoplasty surgeons proceed without marking the nose, a plan having taken form in their "mind's eye." With time, the learning resident surgeon will be able to "see" the anatomy, hidden by overlying skin, between palpating fingers and correctly positioned instruments. Until that time, mark the nasal skin with topographic guides (Fig. 11-5):

Proposed line of dorsal resection
Margins of lower lateral cartilage with proposed resection limits
Line of osteotomy
Extent of alar base excision (when indicated).

Regional Anesthesia

The sensory innervation of the nose is from the supratrochlear nerves in the nasion, infraorbital nerve laterally, the external nasal dorsally (Fig. 11-6) and internally, and the sphenopalatine ganglion internally (Fig. 11-7). Each must be blocked by infiltration or by topical anesthesia.

Begin with adequate sedation. Then soak cotton or Q-tips with 4% cocaine. Place one anteriorly in each nostril to block the mucosal branches of the anterior ethmoid and another for the posterior to block the sphenopalatine ganglion (Fig. 11-8). This one is important; tuck it under the middle turbinate.

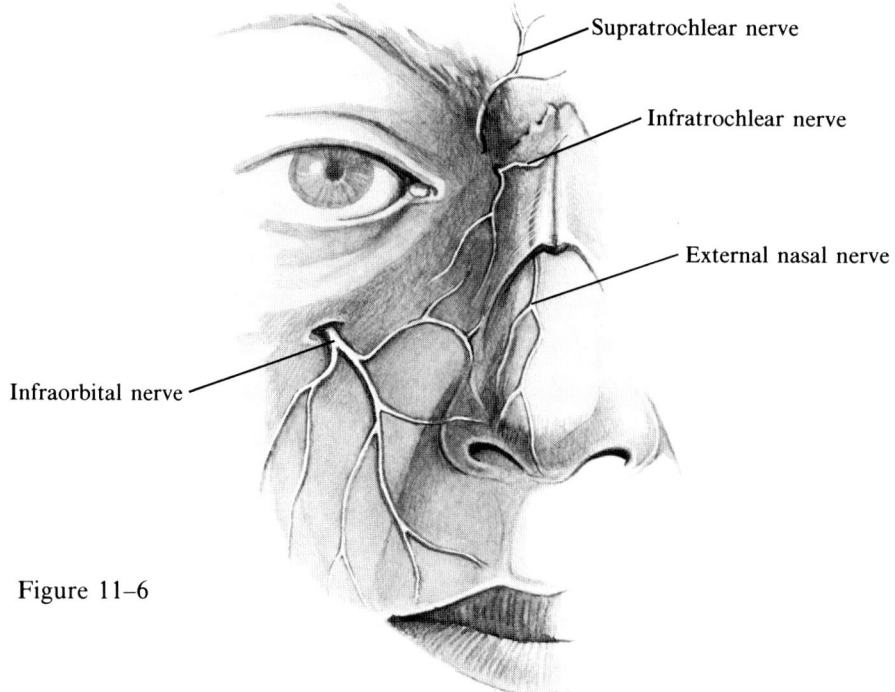

Figure 11-6

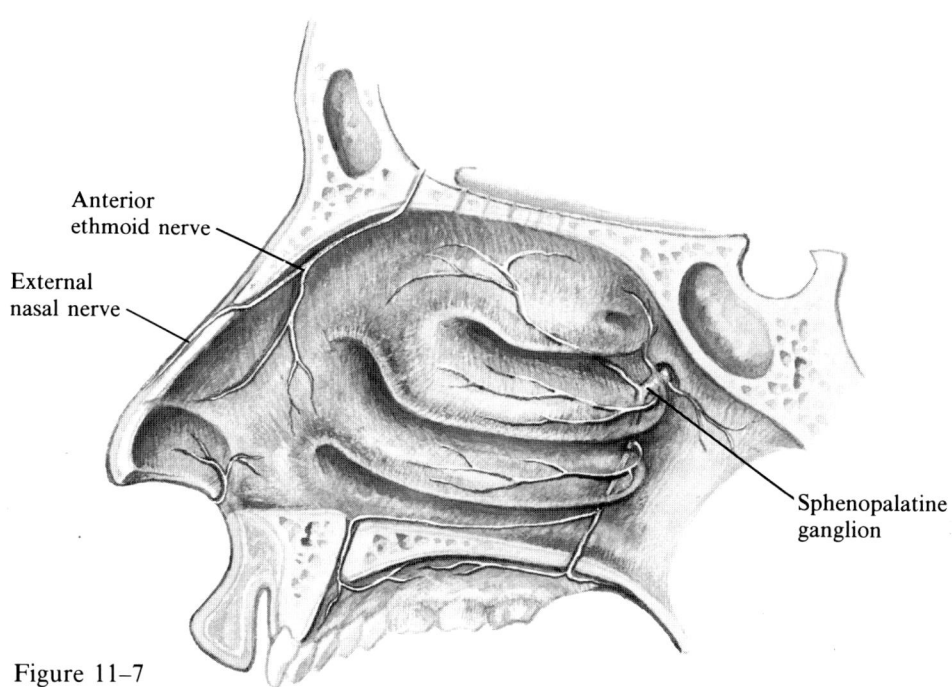

Figure 11-7

A third swab can rest along the nasal floor on each side. Next, infiltrate with 1% or 2% xylocaine, with added epinephrine (1:100,000 or 1:200,000). Use no larger than a 27-gauge needle. Infiltrate the glabellar region, then block the infraorbital nerve beginning at the alar base, fanning out laterally and superiorly toward the infraorbital foramen (Fig. 11-9). Do not insert the needle into the foramen because lasting neural injury may result. Next, block the nasal tip, infiltrating the external nasal branches of the anterior

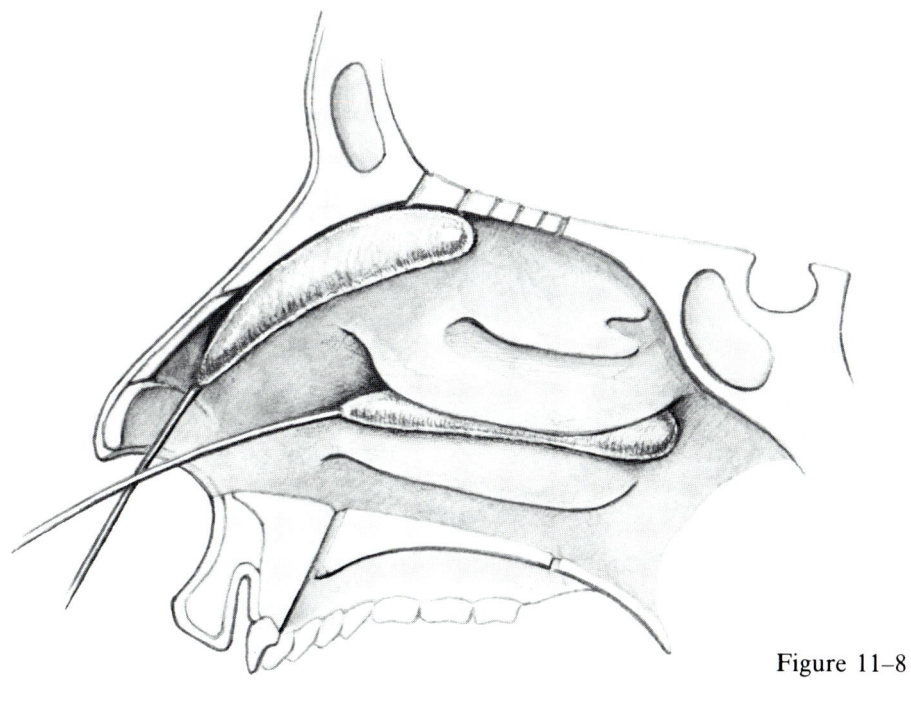

Figure 11-8

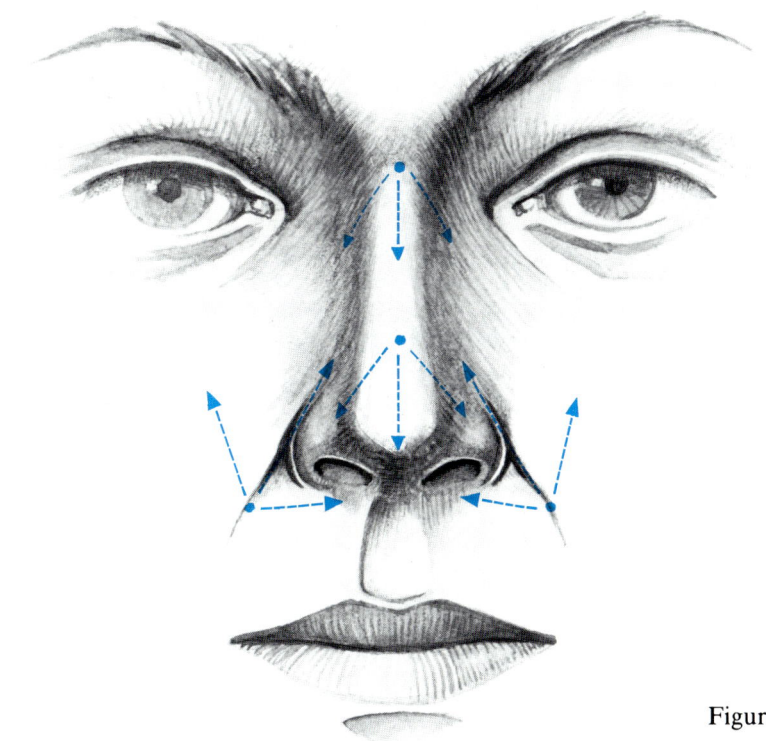

Figure 11-9

ethmoid as they emerge from beneath the upper lateral cartilages. This can also be accomplished from within, injecting between the cartilages. Finally, block the distal palatine branches at the nasal spine. Inject at the base of the columella or into the upper buccal sulcus in midline. This final injection will hurt patients the most. Save it until last. Trim vibrissae (nostril hair) at this time with blunt-nosed scissors. Apply ointment to the scissor tips to catch loose hair. Leave anesthetic packs in nose until after prep and draping.

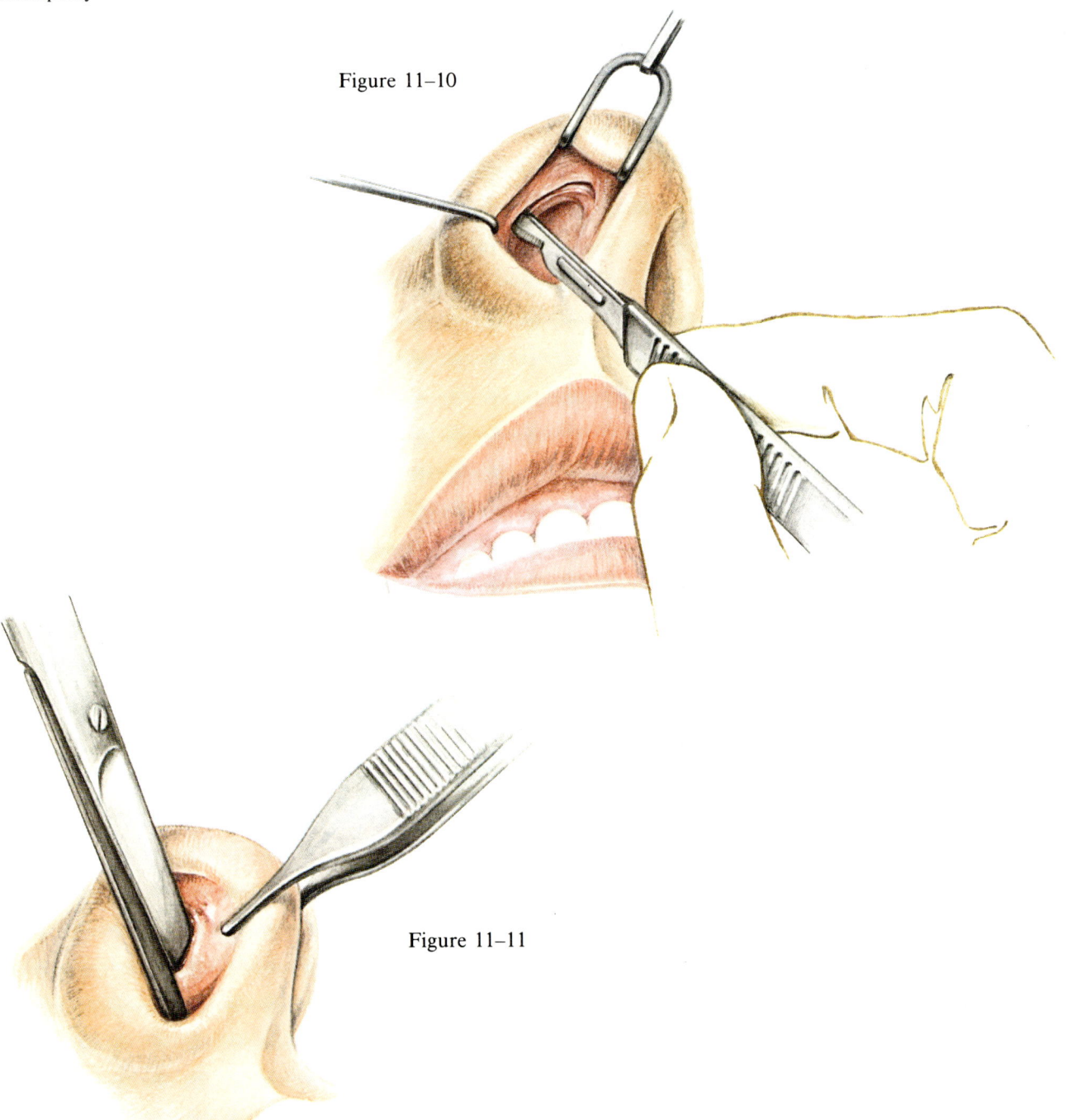

Figure 11–10

Figure 11–11

Operative Technique

1. Retract nostril rim with Foman ball-tipped retractor (Fig. 11–10). Incise with No. 15 blade knife the intracartilaginous mucosa, a hollow visible between retractor and leading edge of upper lateral cartilage. Extend the incision medial to the septum, then curve around angle and several millimeters down the septum.
2. Only if necessary, separate columella from caudal edge of the septum using knife and scissors (the so-called transfixion incision) (Fig. 11–11).
3. Dissect soft tissues free of underlying skeleton with blunt tip scissors (Fig. 11–12). Take care not to dissect laterally anymore than necessary to reduce dorsum. Otherwise, nasal bones will fall inward after osteotomy. Complete this step by lifting periosteum off bony dorsum with a Joseph elevator (Fig. 11–13).
4. Reduce nasal bridge to predetermined level with diamond-type rasp, avoid separation of upper lateral cartilage from bony dorsum (Fig. 11–14).

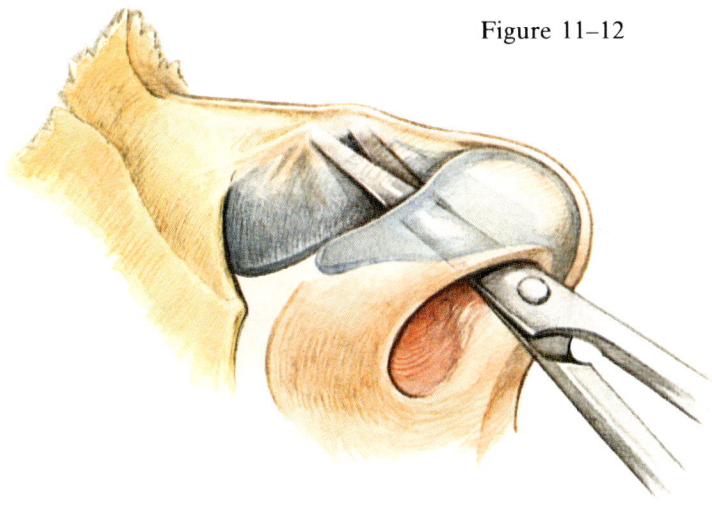

Figure 11–12

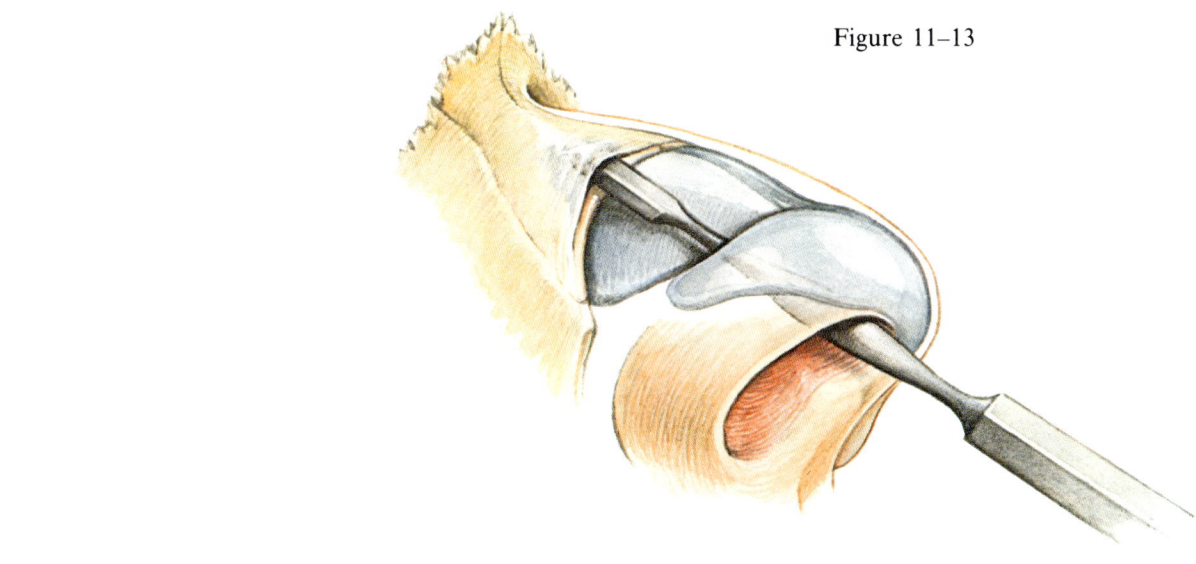

Figure 11–13

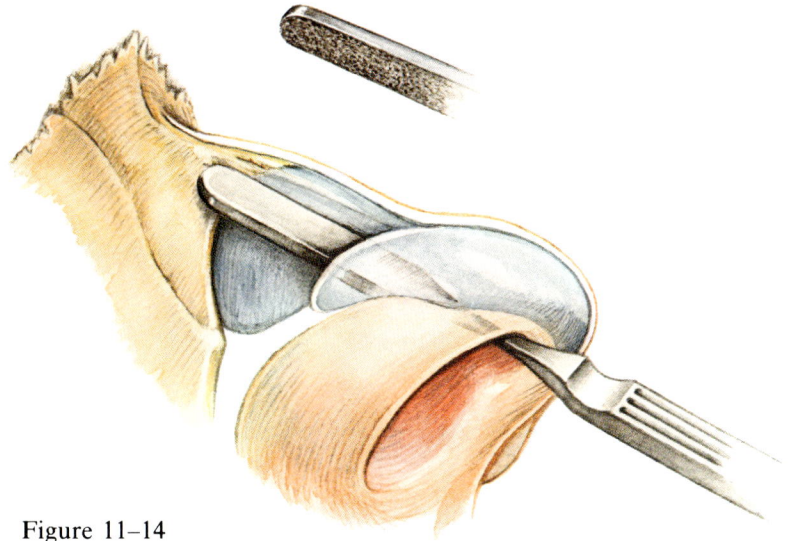

Figure 11–14

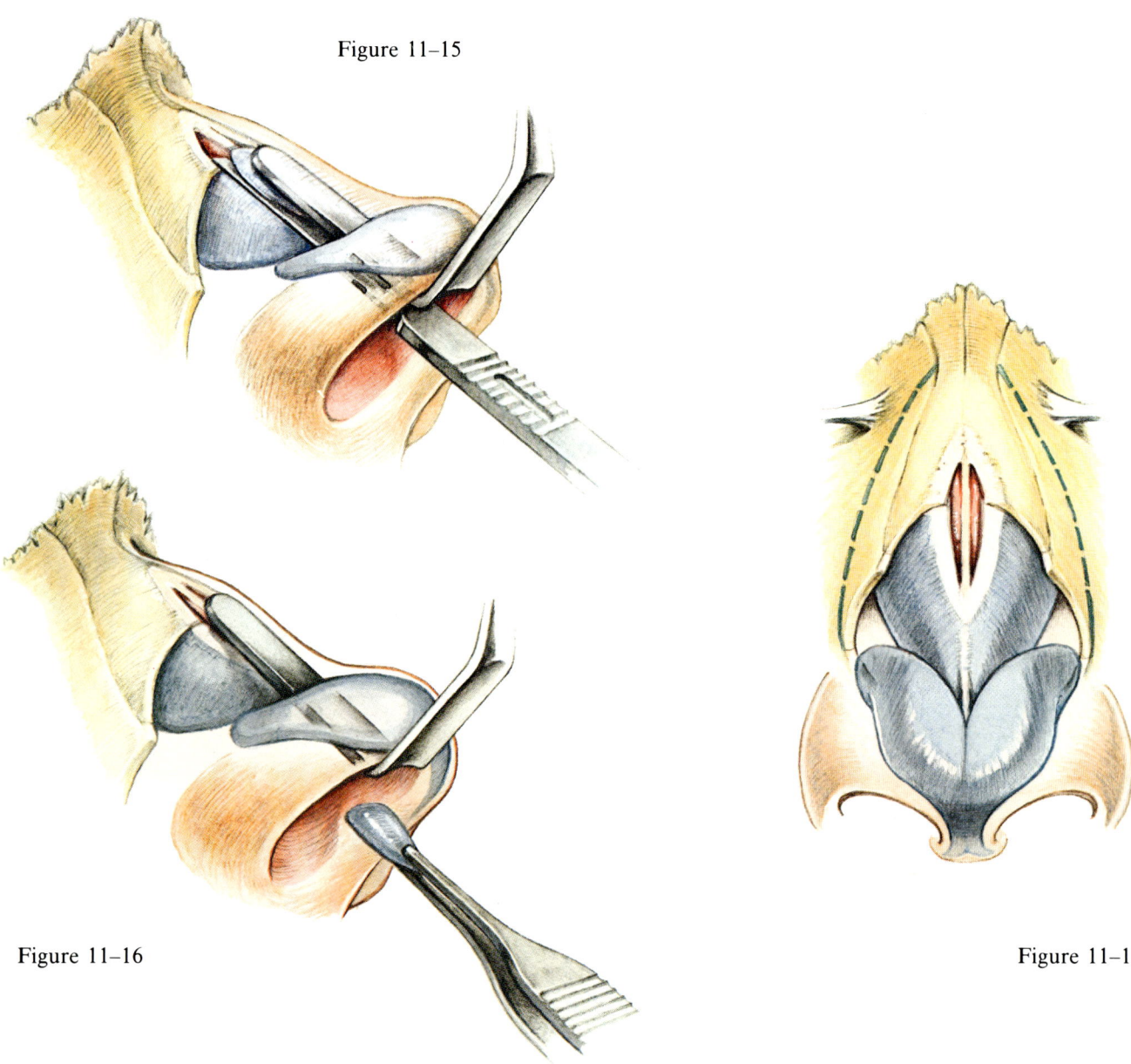

Figure 11-15

Figure 11-16

Figure 11-17

5. Insert long-bladed Auficht retractor into the intercartilaginous incision. Complete bridge reduction by trimming septum and upper lateral cartilages with No. 11 blade (sans tip), matching cartilage to bone for desired profile. If possible, leave the nasal mucosa intact (Figs. 11-15 and 11-16).
6. Smooth entire dorsum with rasp. Remove fragments of cartilage and bone under direct vision.
7. Nasal osteotomies are indicated if the bony pyramid is wide or deviated, or if the roof is open (meaning a significant gap between nasal bones (Fig. 11-17). Osteotomies can be done with saws or osteotomies or a combination of the two. Begin with a perforating incision using a No. 15 blade in the nasal vestibule at the base of the nasal pyramid. Advance knife to bone edge, establishing a tract for the Joseph elevator. Insert elevator to free periosteum from osteotomy site. You can weaken bone first with saw or begin with an osteotome. Begin low, end high on bone. An experienced assistant must guide you. At this point, direct osteotome with one hand, feel course of tip with other, and ask assistant to wield

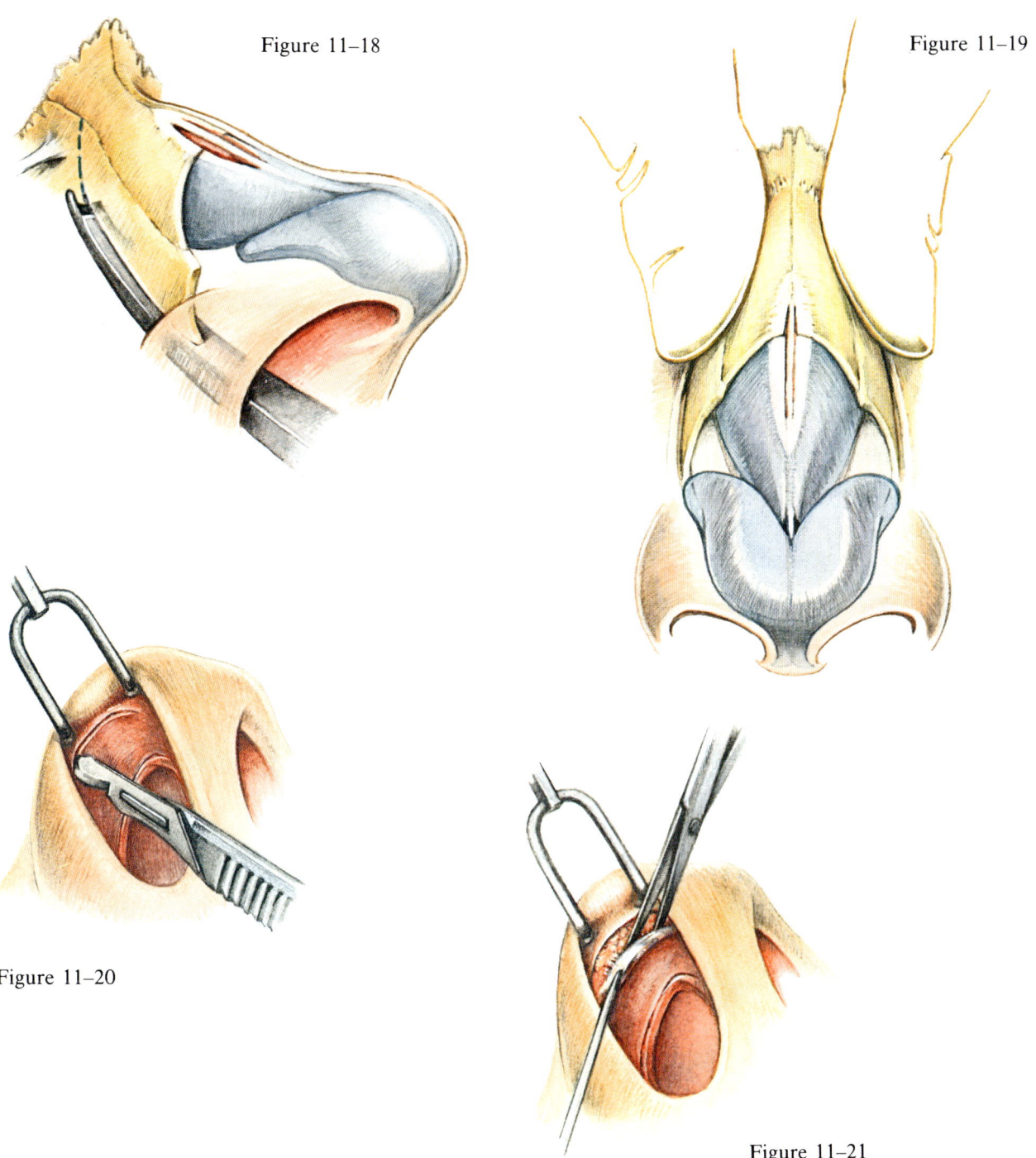

Figure 11–18

Figure 11–19

Figure 11–20

Figure 11–21

the mallet, pausing briefly after each two strikes. Stay forward of medial canthal ligament as osteotome is advanced superiorly. Listen for change in tone when osteotome reaches the glabella (Fig. 11–18).

8. Complete fracture with fingers; bone should "greenstick" at nasion (Fig. 11–19). If not, insert 1–2 mm osteotome through overlying skin to complete fracture. The bridge is complete: focus now on the tip.

9. Make a "rim" incision in the skin just inside the nostril border (Fig. 11–20). It should be distal to the previous intracartilaginous incision and sufficiently long to allow lower lateral cartilage to be brought out into direct view as a bipedicle flap of cartilage and vestibular lining. Free the cartilage from overlying skin using a Stephens tenotomy scissors (Fig. 11–21). Alar rim is retracted superiorly, the bipedicle flap inferiorly with skin hook.

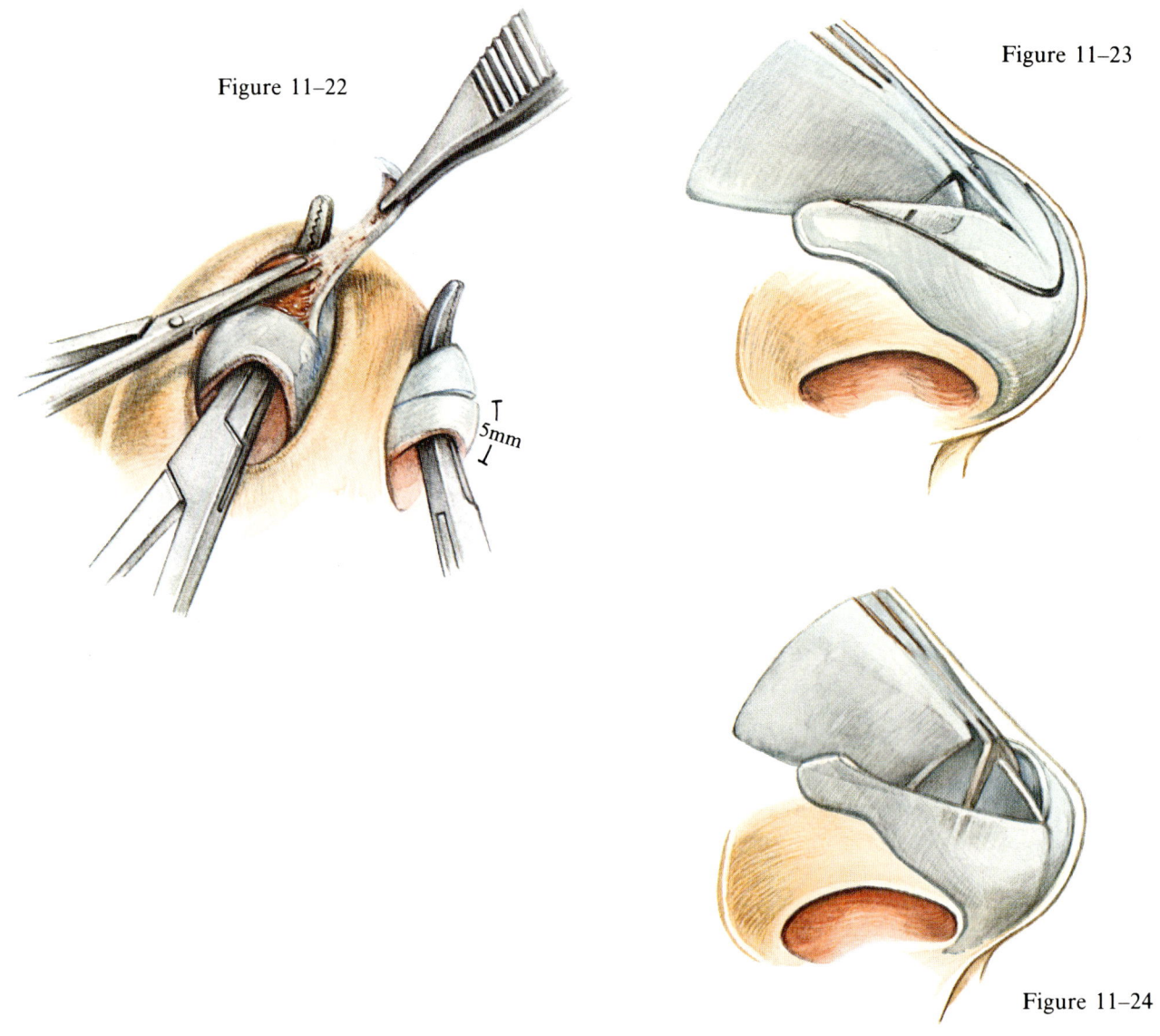

Figure 11-22

Figure 11-23

Figure 11-24

10. With a scalpel, mark cartilage to be left intact (4–5 mm). Trim remaining cartilage from the cephalic border but *leave all lining intact* (Fig. 11-22). Extend cartilage excision over dome medially. Return flap to anatomic position and check tip contour. Sculpture further as necessary.
11. Evaluate dorsum–tip relationship. Tip should now be rotated superiorly, increasing the nasolabial angle. Lower lateral cartilages should rise above level of dorsum. Also examine relationship of ala to the columella and the nasolabial angle (Figs. 11-23 and 11-24).
12. Make necessary alterations in tip–bridge relationship now. Trim caudal septum as needed. Correct obtuse nasolabial angle by resecting nasal spine. Consider at this time tip augmentation with cartilage grafts.
13. Now reconstruct the internal valve. Because the tip has rotated upward superiorly, the distal upper lateral cartilage will project caudal to the new interval valve determined by the intercartilaginous incision. Dissect this cartilage from the lining and shorten it, preserving all mucosa.

14. Close rim incisions with 5-0 chromic sutures. Close transfixion incision, if present, with 4-0 absorbable sutures, positioning them to establish appropriate columella position.
15. Suction any clot from the dorsal space. Irrigate if necessary, and insert a very small pack of lubricated gauze in the nostril to help support incision and prevent adhesions. Do not pack nose tightly; avoid distracting nasal bones.
16. Tape dorsum with ½ inch adhesive tape. Mold tip with tape. Apply dorsal plaster cast extending from glabella to supratip region. The splint remains for 5-7 days. Supplement with easily removable and absorbent gauze at the tip to collect drainage.

Variations

The principal goal of this chapter is description of a basic sequence for corrective rhinoplasty. A single "best" way does not exist. There are many variations, some of them merely alternate ways to achieve an identical goal. For example:

Alternate Osteotomy Methods
Joseph relied on a saw to first weaken, then fracture the nasal pyramid. Today, osteotomies are more popular. Some surgeons still weaken the bone or establish tracks in the bone with a saw, then insert an osteotome to complete fracture. Others introduce a narrow (2 mm) osteotome through a tiny percutaneous wound medial to each inner canthus, making multiple bony perforations along desired fracture line that permits easy infracturing.

Airway Obstruction
This may be due to septal deviation, turbinate hypertrophy or vomerine spur enlargement. Solutions include resection of offending cause, perhaps septum and/or turbinate.

Deviated Nose
The asymmetric bony pyramid is corrected by osteotomy. Associated septal malposition requires individualized treatment depending on circumstance, perhaps a hinged mucoperichondral flap or scoring of cartilage (Septoplasty).

Lack of Tip Projection
Use of cartilage grafts to ensure tip projections has been popularized by Sheen.

Broad or Ultra (Pinocchio) Tip
Purposeful use of complete transfixion incision together with scoring of lateral cartilages or removal of lateral crus serves to deemphasize exaggerated tip.

Saddle Nose Deformity
This may be congenital or caused by trauma, or be secondary to overzealous rhinoplasty. It requires for solution the use of septal or conchal grafts of cartilage, and in severe cases, an L-shaped bone graft.

Alar Deformity
Flaring nostrils can be tailored by alar base excision (Weir wedges). Read Millard on this problem.

Chin Recession
Restoration of facial balance may require use of chin implant at the time of rhinoplasty.

Issues

As stated earlier in this volume, certain controversies are given the appearance of genuine issues when in fact they are only variations. Some attach importance to the following "issues:"

Tip First/Dorsum First
Sheen and others assign importance to reducing the dorsum first, then matching tip to bridge. Peck, on the other hand, advocates tip sculpturing first, then matching bridge to tip. Close examination of the superior results of each proves that both approaches can be applied successfully.

Outfracture and/or Infracture
Some stress importance of "outfracturing nasal pyramid" whereas others say that instability can follow vigorous handling of bone fragments, leading to excessive narrowing of bridge.

Transfixion Incision
Complete separation of the columella from the septum, once routine, is now suspect. Critics maintain that the inevitable contraction of the scar contributes to postoperative tip depression. Some resist transfixion incisions, citing their lack of necessity unless the nasal spine must be resected. Even then, exposure can be achieved without extending the incision to the columellar base.

Dorsal Resection
Some advocate additional resection of dorsum to compensate for inevitable tip drop after surgery. Others caution against this habit. "Ill advised," they say; better to perceive the constricted tip and achieve a solution with tip grafts.

Valve Interruption
Separation of lower lateral cartilages from septum, traditional in some hands, creates valve malfunction say others, and is entirely unnecessary say another camp.

Additional Reading

Natvig P. Jacques Joseph—Surgical Sculptor. Saunders, Philadelphia, 1982.
Aufricht G. Rhinoplasty and the face. Plast Reconstr Surg 43:219, 1969.
Dingman RO and Natvig P. Surgical anatomy in aesthetic and corrective rhinoplasty. Clin Past Surg 4:111, 1977.
Sheen JH. Aesthetic Rhinoplasty. C.V. Mosby, St. Louis, 1978.
Peck G. The difficult nasal tip. Clin Plast Surg 4:103, 1977.
Millard DR. Secondary corrective rhinoplasty. Plast Reconstr Surg 44:545, 1969.
Rees TR. Current concepts of rhinoplasty. Clin Plast Surg 4:131, 1977.
Rees TD. Aesthetic Plastic Surgery, Volume 1. Saunders, Philadelphia, 1980. (Entire first volume of this two volume encyclopedia reference deals with rhinoplasty in fine detail.)

Dermabrasion, Chemical Peel, and Collagen Injection

David H. Frank and Leonard W. Glass

Associated with aesthetic facial procedures such a facelift, blepharoplasty, and rhinoplasty, are three techniques used to enhance the results of surgery. They are chemical peel, dermabrasion, and collagen injection, each one an adjunct measure for hiding irregularities of skin surface texture. Frown lines, acne scars, posttraumatic scars, various soft tissue contour deformities resulting from congenital deformity, trauma, infection, or aging may all benefit from these techniques.

Surgeons who recognize opportunities for these adjunctive methods should propose their use to patients *before surgery,* so they can be viewed as a planned supplementary step rather than as secondary correction of surgery already performed.

Indications for these measures overlap. Their application must be considered by both surgeon and patient just as carefully as any surgical undertaking. They may appear simple, but skill and judgement are required, as complications can be extraordinarily deforming.

Dermabrasion

Dermabrasion is a controlled abrasive technique for planing an irregular skin surface. Dermabrasion stimulates inflammation but not as deeply as does chemical peeling. Recovery is therefore faster, erythema less intense, risk of hyperpigmentation less pronounced, but the degree of improvement less obvious.

Indications (Fig. 12-1)

1. Acne scars: Dermabrasion was first advocated decades ago; it is still in use, but is not nearly as effective as reported in the lay press. Only 25-30% of pitted acneiform scars are shallow enough to benefit from dermabrasion. But this seems enough to please most patients.
2. Circumoral wrinkles: Those fine radial lines about the mouth will be more conspicuous after facelift. They can be made less apparent by dermabrasion done at the same time as facelift.
3. Scars: Some small irregular scars can be improved by dermabrasion, but do not rely on this method for most scars. Remember that scars are made of collagen, not of skin. Abrasion stimulates inflammation and therefore induces more collagen synthesis.

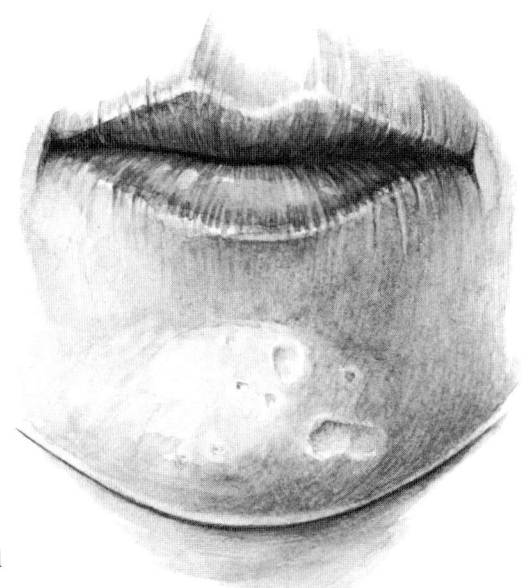

Figure 12–1

4. Overgrafting: The epithelium can be dermabraded from atrophic or color mismatched skin grafts, providing a wound base that accepts a better quality skin graft.

Contraindications

1. Patients with "olive"-hued skin or those already displaying hyperpigmentation are *not* good prospects for dermabrasion. More striking hyperpigmentation may be encountered by these individuals.
2. Burn scars are densely collagenous and only minor irregularities of an epithelial surface can be occasionally improved following dermabrasion.
3. Patients taking exogenous estrogen are more likely to develop hyperpigmentation after dermabrasion.

What the Patient Needs to Know Before the Procedure

1. Following dermabrasion, fine-mesh gauze will be placed on the wound and allowed to dry. An outer absorbant dressing will be changed or removed after the first day.
2. After 5 days, a water-based ointment is applied several times daily to the gauze, which loosens with water soaks and is removed over several days. The skin beneath will be pink and will remain so for 4–8 weeks. Cosmetics may be used 3–5 days after epithelialization is complete. Restrict sun exposure for several weeks.
3. Hypopigmentation can be expected in dermabraded zones.
4. Frequent complications include persistent itching and early hyperpigmentation.
5. Less common complications include persistent hyperpigmentation, full thickness skin loss, and scars (whenever safe depth is exceeded).

Regional Anesthesia

Infiltrate at subdermal level all zones to be dermabraded, with 1% xylocaine and 1:100,000 epineprine.

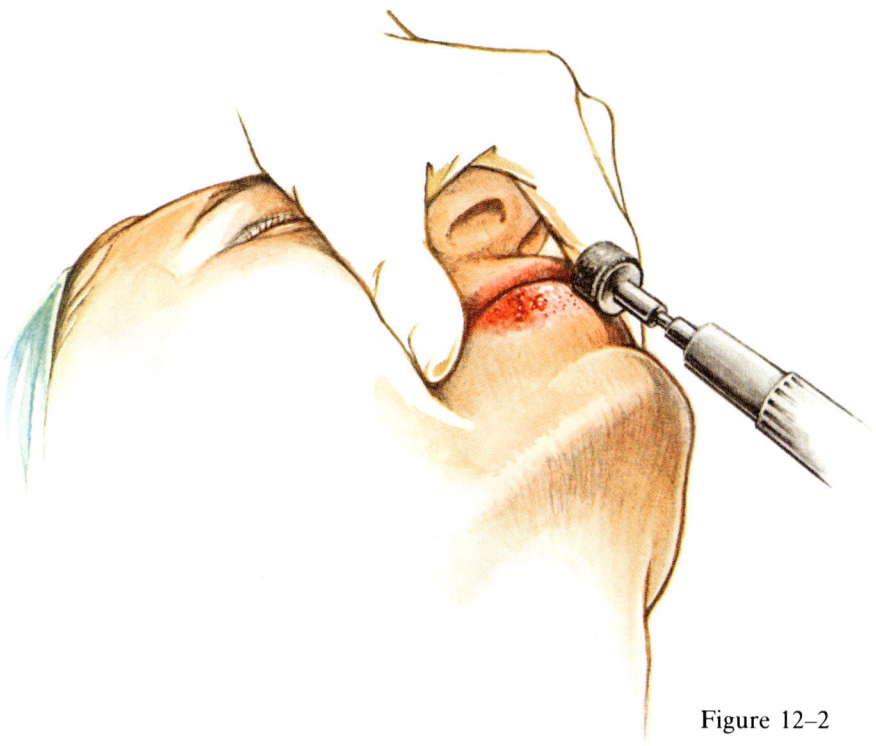

Figure 12–2

Technique

We prefer to use a wire brush wheel instead of a diamond-tipped brush or other device. Prep patient and drape carefully and tightly, leaving no loose ends or sponges near field. Hold dermabrador in one hand, apply skin tension with the other (Fig. 12–2). Move wheel over skin, applying even pressure over the entire zone. Stop when punctate bleeding sites appear in the dermis. Then move on to the next zone. An assistant can maintain a moist surface with light saline irrigation. Make certain that symmetric zones are dermabraded on each side. Around the mouth, abrade across the skin-vermillion border, and onto the lip. Be most cautious near the eyes. An assistant must protect globe and eyelids with a tongue blade.

Apply an impregnated gauze (e.g., Xeroform). Supplement with absorptive dressings if desired. Remove all but inner gauze at 24 h. Remove all dressings by the sixth day.

Chemical Peel

A chemical peel is limited to the face and is synonymous with "face peel." Consider this technique as a controlled destruction of the outer skin layers following inflammation and microscopic necrosis. The healing process that follows is a subtle contraction of the healing skin, followed by diminished prominence of wrinkles.

Indications

1. An adjunct to a surgical facelift, but *rarely if ever* a substitute for facelift. Only the most shallow skin creases will be improved.

2. Diffuse acne scarring.
3. Used very infrequently to counteract hyperpigmentation following use of birth control pills ("mask of pregnancy").

Contraindications

1. Patients with a history of heart disease or antiarrhythmic medications.
2. Patients with "olive"-hued or other heavily pigmented skin. Hypopigmentation is inevitable after chemical peel, and is all the more evident in well-pigmented skin.
3. Patients who have had facial surgery, especially a facelift, less than 60 days prior. Only perioral peeling can be safely done at the same time as a facelift.
4. Patients with healed skin grafts or healed partial thickness facial burns should *never* be peeled.
5. Patients taking exogenous estrogen are more likely to develop hyperpigmentation.

What the Patient Needs to Know Before the Procedure

1. A chemical peel works by destroying the outer layers of the skin. After healing, the skin is thinner and less elastic.
2. Loss of skin pigment after chemical peeling is inevitable.
3. Wait at least 2 months after a facelift before scheduling a chemical peel. Then limit direct sun exposure 2–4 additional months.
4. Pain can be a prominent feature following a chemical peel. Narcotic analgesia will be prescribed. The pain passes in 24–48 h.
5. Ask patient to take oral fluids to assist phenol excretion.
6. Heart beat irregularities are to be reported promptly to the surgeon.
7. The face will be taped after peeling. It is removed 48 h afterward. A medicated powder (e.g., thymol iodide) can be applied to absorb inflammatory exudate. (This is an uncomfortable time for the patient.)
8. A shower 5 days after peeling helps remove the accumulated facial crusts.
9. An antibiotic ointment may be applied after each daily shower for a week or so.
10. The face will be red. This fades in 2–4 months. Use of moisturizing cream is appropriate during this interval. Makeup can be used after crusts fall off.
11. Itching can be an annoyance for several days or weeks after peeling.
12. Uncommon complications include skin loss, scars, contraction/distortion, asymmetry, or skip areas.

What the Surgeon Needs to Know

1. Phenol (carbolic acid) is the active agent in the peeling solution and is a very effective coagulator of protein. Be certain it is prepared carefully by the pharmacist. Do not splash the solution in the eye (patient's or surgeon's). Protect fingers with gloves while handling solution.
2. Phenol solution is 50% and is mixed as follows:
   3 ml phenol
   2 ml distilled water
   3 drops croton oil
   8 drops liquid soap
   Mix all ingredients and wait 60 min.

3. Skin can absorb significant quantities of phenol. Systemic complications include paroxysmal atrial tachycardia, central nervous system irritability and seizures, hemolysis, and renal tubular necrosis. Therefore, maintain sedation, hydrate, and *apply the solution very slowly.*

Regional Anesthesia

Xylocaine infiltration is not needed but analgesia and sedation are; they counteract central nervous system irritability induced by the absorbed phenol as well as minimize the burning sensation following application. *Use of xylocaine and epinephrine is discouraged because they can extend depth of chemical wound.*

Technique

1. Mix solution yourself or obtain it freshly prepared from a reliable source. Allow it to sit 1 h before application.
2. Remove surface skin oils with ether (acetone is acceptable if ether is unavailable).
3. Take at least 60 min to apply the solution to the entire face. Rapid application of phenol increases risk of paroxysmal atrial tachycardia. Therefore, divide face into thirds; apply phenol, then tape before going on to the next zone. Take 20 min for forehead and eyelids, an equivalent period for the nose, lips and chin, and finally 20 min more to complete the cheeks.
4. Apply solution evenly. Stir or shake solution frequently throughout the procedure. Saturate cotton-tipped applicator; then squeeze out surplus inside the neck of the bottle. Stroke skin with Q-tips while other hand passes over the surface with a cotton ball to ensure even application (Fig. 12–3).

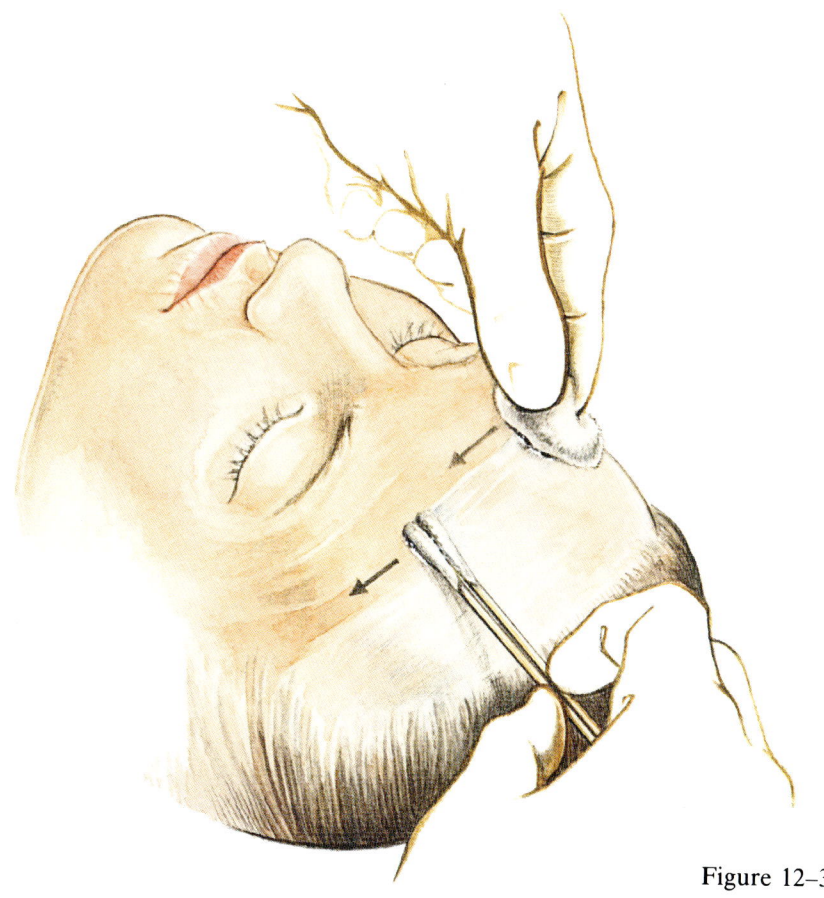

Figure 12–3

Dermabrasion, Chemical Peel, and Collagen Injection

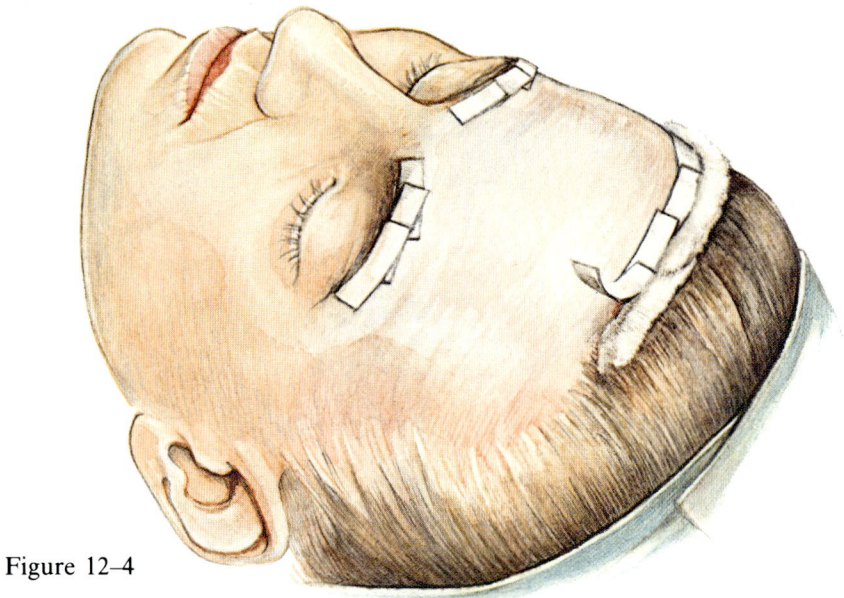

Figure 12–4

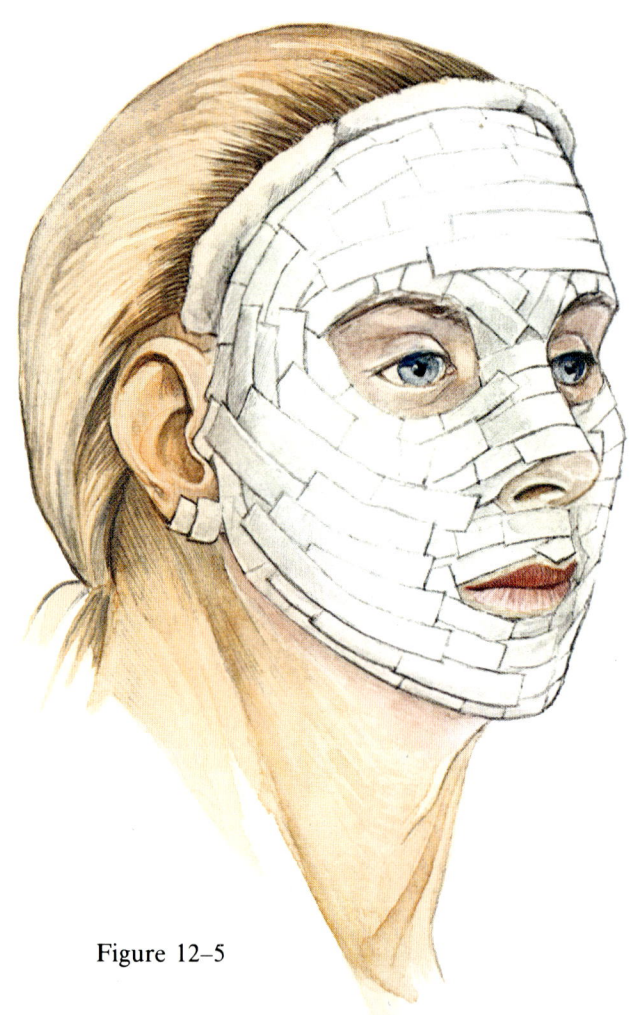

Figure 12–5

118

5. Apply solution well into hairline to avoid sharp demarcation lines. Apply solution to upper lids down to palpebral fold, and to lower lids up to within 1 mm of lashes. Do not apply solution in the hollow above or medial to the inner canthus; contraction bands may develop.
6. Do the columella along with the nose. Do not omit the earlobes. When applying solution to the lips, go onto the vermillion slightly.
7. In the cheek region, extend application 1 cm inferior to the mandibular margin, feathering lightly into the unpeeled zone. Do not tape this feathered zone. Demarcation will also be hidden by the natural shadow.
8. Waterproof adhesive tape (½ inch) is applied to all peeled zones for retention of heat and extension of the depth of injury. Omit tape from eyelids. Protect hairline with cotton when applying the tape so removal will be less painful (Figs. 12–4 and 12–5).

Collagen Injection

As of this writing, the jury is still out on the usefulness of injectible collagen as an adjunct to surgery of the aging face. One fact is clear, however; collagen is far safer than liquid silicone and should in time supplant hazards of silicone use.

Problems associated with clinical use of liquid silicone relate to impurities of the material injected, or to misapplication in body regions other than the face. Because liquid silicone is so tissue-nonreactive, it is prone to migration within tissue planes. At present, high-grade dimethyl polysiloxane is manufactured by Dow-Corning and is registered as an investigational material for use only in the facial region.

Only injectable collagen (Zyderm® by Collagen Corporation) has earned FDA approval for clinical use; the following discussion is therefore limited to collagen.

Indications

Zyderm® seems best suited for augmentation of soft tissue depressions in soft distensible lesions with smooth margins. These include:

1. Acne scars
2. Localized steroid atrophy
3. Glabellar furrows
4. Postrhinoplasty irregularities
5. Depressed traumatic scars
6. Depressed skin grafts
7. Lipodystrophy.

Lesions with sharp borders or nondistensible scars are less likely to benefit from collagen.

Contraindications

1. Previous injection of liquid silicone
2. Family history of autoimmune or rheumatic diseases
3. Known allergic reaction to lidocaine
4. Adverse reaction to Zyderm® skin test
5. Zyderm® is *not approved* for use in breast, bone, tendon, ligament, or muscle tissue.

What the Patient Needs to Know Before the Procedure

1. Collagen (Zyderm®) is a newly approved product. Although it appears safe, long-term side effects are as yet unknown.
2. Several injections may be necessary.
3. The "final" correction after one or more injections is *not* permanent. Repeat touch ups are likely to be required at intervals of 6 months to 2 years to maintain level of correction.
4. Collagen does not replace standard surgical procedures. It is an adjunctive technique.
5. Following injection, there will be temporary over correction; swelling and redness should subside within 24–48 h. Report to your surgeon any itching. Increased swelling, or redness.
6. Adverse (allergic) reactions, infection, and reactivation or herpes simplex have all been reported.
7. Sun exposure and alcohol consumption have resulted in localized reaction at the injection site.

What the Surgeon Must Know

1. Injectible collagen (Zyderm®) is a highly purified bovine dermal collagen. A portion of the protein molecule has been enzymatically removed to diminish antigenicity. Zyderm® is suspended in physiologic saline and 0.3% lidocaine. Following injection, saline is absorbed, leaving a soft cohesive implant 25–30% of the original volume. Host cells are said to invade the implanted protein, making it a "viable" tissue replacement although this has not been established.
2. FDA restricts Zyderm® use to 30 ml per patient per year. A defect requiring more volume should be treated by other means.
3. Best level for injection is intradermal or in the superficial subdermal tissue plane.
4. Overcorrection by factor of 1.5–2× defect will yield best result and diminish need to reinject.

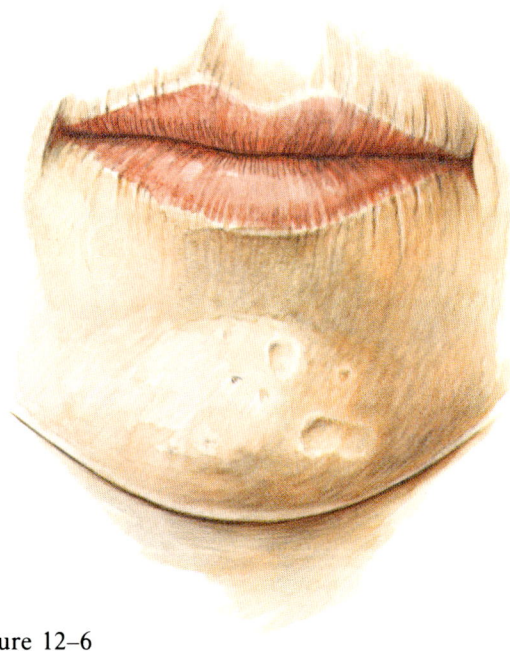

Figure 12–6

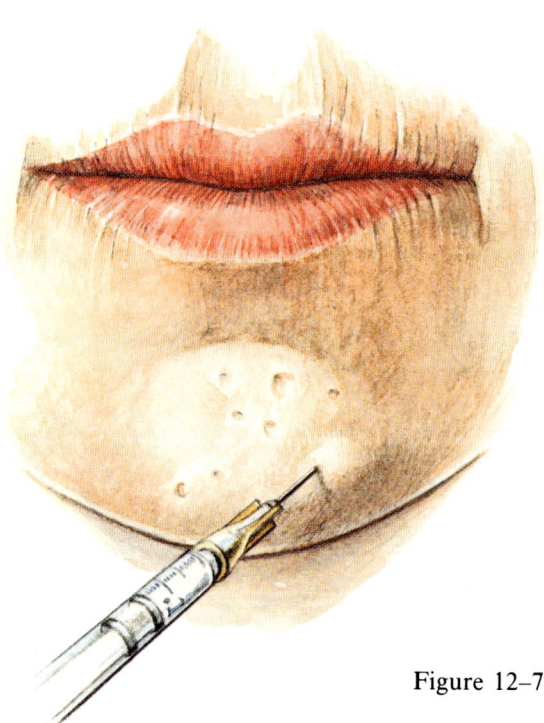

Figure 12–7

5. Overcorrections in periorbital or vermillion zones are slow to resolve; caution is advised.
6. For scars, inject within, but not beneath.
7. Zyderm® injection can be combined with dermabrasion; inject first, abrade later.

Technique

1. Skin test: 0.1 cc Zyderm® given intradermally, volar forearm. Site is observed 4 weeks for reaction. There is 3% incidence of test site reactivity.
2. After skin prep, inject through 27-gauge needle, remaining within scar, or in dermis, overcorrecting 1.5–2 times depth of lesion (Figs. 12–6 and 12–7).
3. Repeat injections at 2-week or longer intervals until adequate correction is achieved.

Variations

Zyderm II® has recently been released with the claim that it produces quicker, more lasting results than Zyderm I®. It is the same modified protein packaged in a higher concentration so that for a given volume more "active" agent and less water is deposited. Experience is too limited to substantiate these claims of increased efficacy.

Additional Reading

Baker TJ. Chemical face peeling and rhytidoplasty. Plast Reconstr Surg 29:199, 1962.

Litton C. Chemical face lifting. Plast Reconstr Surg 29:371–380, 1962. (These two articles are among the first appearing in the Plastic Surgery literature discribing the indications, techniques, and complications of chemical peels. The cautious, documented approach of the second article is particularly worth reading.)

Baker TJ and Gordon HL. Chemical face peeling and dermabrasion. Surg Clin North Am 51:387–401, 1971. (Describes the indications for these two procedures and compares their results.)

Spira M, Gerow F, and Hardy SB. Complications of chemical face peeling. Plast Reconstr Surg 54:397–403, 1974. (A must read article for anyone contemplating doing chemical peeling.)

Knapp TR, Luck E, and Daniels JR. Injectable collagen for soft tissue augmentation. Plast Reconstr Surg 60:398–405, 1977. (One of the first reports by the developers of injectable collagen. Discusses its biochemical properties and potential clinical uses.)

Zyderm collagen implant. Med Lett Drugs Ther 24(614):69–70, 1982. (A very brief, unbiased summary of the use of injectable collagen.)

Kaplan EN, Falces E, and Tolleth H. Clinical utilization of injectable collagen. Ann Plast Surg 10:437–451, 1983. (These authors present their experience in 400 patients over a 6-year period. Indications for its use and extensive photographs are presented optimistically.)

Swanson NA, Stoner JG, Siegle RJ, et al. Treatment site reactions to Zyderm collagen implantation. J Dermatol Surg Oncol 9:377–380, 1983. (Local complications following use of injectable collagen are presented and should be reviewed prior to using the material for the first time.)

Cohen IK, Peacock EE, Chvapil M. Zyderm, Letter to the Editor. Plast Reconstr Surg 73:857–858, 1984. (Thoughtful plastic surgeons, knowleadgable in the field of collagen biochemistry, who raise important issues of long term safety.)

Index

Abdominoplasty, 39–49
  anesthesia for, 41
  background to, 39
  choice of incisions, 48
  contraindications to, 39
  electrocautery vs. knife dissection, 49
  indications for, 39
  operative planning, 41
  operative technique, 43–48
  patient information prior to, 40
  surgeon information prior to, 40–41
  variations in, 48–49
Acne scars, dermabrasion for, 113
Aesthetic indications, for breast reduction/elevation, 25
Aesthetic surgeon, education of, 1–3
Aesthetic surgery
  day of, 11
  patient selection for, 5–8
  preparation prior to, 10
  sedation for, 9–12
Airway obstruction, 111
Alar deformity, 111
Anesthesia
  for abdominoplasty, 41
  for breast reduction/elevation, 29
  for facelift, 64
  for forehead lift, 88
  regional, 16
    for blepharoplasty, 54
    for chemical peel, 117
    for dermabrasion, 114
    for necklift, 79
    for rhinoplasty, 103–105
Anxiety, preoperative, 11
Augmentation mammaplasty, 13–23
  background to, 13
  contraindications to, 14–15
  controversy associated with, 23
  indications for, 13–14
  operative design, 16
  operative technique, 16–21
  patient information prior to, 15
  periareolar incision for, 22
  postoperative care, 20
  subpectoral implantation, 22–23
  surgeon information prior to, 15
  variations in, 22–23

Blepharoplasty, 51–57
  background to, 51
  and browlift, 57
  contraindications to, 51–52
  indications for, 51
  issues in, 57
  operative planning, 53
  operative technique, 54–56
  patient information prior to, 52
  surgeon information prior to, 52–53
  variations in, 56
Blood supply
  to face, 63
  to nipple, 27
Breast disease, screening for, 27
Breast flap design, variations in, 37
Breast reduction/elevation, 25–38
  anesthesia for, 29
  background to, 25
  contraindications to, 26
  indications for, 25
  issues in, 38
  operative design, 28–29
  operative technique, 30–35
  patient information prior to, 26–27
  surgeon information prior to, 27
  variations in, 36–37
Breasts, enlargement of, see Augmentation mammaplasty
Breast topography, 27
Browlift, blepharoplasty and, 57

Brow prominence, lateral, correction of, 56

Chemical peel, 115–118
  contraindications to, 116
  indications for, 115–116
  patient information prior to, 116
  regional anesthesia for, 117
  surgeon information prior to, 116–117
  technique, 117–118
Chin recession, 112
Cocaine, for rhinoplasty, 103–104
Collagen injection, 118–121
  contraindications to, 119
  indications for, 118–119
  patient information prior to, 119–120
  surgeon information prior to, 120
  technique, 121
  variations in, 121

Dermabrasion, 113–115
  contraindications to, 114
  indications for, 113–114
  patient information prior to, 114
  regional anesthesia for, 114
  technique, 115
Deviated nose, 111
Diazepam (Valium), 11
Dorsal resection, in rhinoplasty, 112
Drugs, for sedation, 11

Ectropion, avoiding, 56
Education, of aesthetic surgeon, 1–3
Electrocautery, vs. knife dissection, for abdominoplasty, 49
Epinephrine, 16
  for blepharoplasty, 54
  for breast reduction/elevation, 29
  for dermabrasion, 114

Index

Epinephrine (*cont.*)
  for facelift, 64
  for rhinoplasty, 104
Eyelids, blepharoplasty of
  lower, 55–56
  upper, 54–55

Face, blood supply to, 63
Facelift, 59–73
  anesthesia for, 64
  background to, 59
  contraindications to, 59–60
  indications for, 59
  issues of, 71–72
  male, 69
  neck incision, 70
  operative design, 63–64
  operative technique, 64–68
  preauricular incision, 70
  patient information prior to, 60–61
  surgeon information prior to, 61–63
  temple incision, 69–70
  variations in, 69–70
Face peel, *see* Chemical peel
Facial nerve, branches of, 62
Facial paralysis, postoperative, 63
Financial transactions, 10
Forehead lift, 85–98
  anesthesia for, 88
  background to, 85
  contraindications to, 85–86
  indications for, 85
  issues in, 96–98
  in men, 96
  operative design, 88
  operative technique, 89–95
  patient information prior to, 86
  surgeon information prior to, 86–87
  variations in, 95–96
Forehead skin excision, direct, 96–97
Frown excision, direct, 97–98

Galea, 86
"Greenstick fracture," 109
Gull-winged coronal incision, 95

Hyperplasia, orbicularis muscle, 56

Implants, for augmentation mammaplasty, 22
Incisions, *see specific types*
Infracture, in rhinoplasty, 112

Knife dissection, vs. electrocautery, for abdominoplasty, 49

Lip, lower, pseudopalsy of, 63

Mammaplasty, augmentation, *see* Augmentation mammaplasty
Mastopexy, *see* Breast reduction/elevation
Medical indications, for breast reduction/elevation, 25
Men
  facelift in, 69
  forehead lift in, 96

Nasal osteotomy, 108
Neck deformity(ies), anatomic classification of, 75
Neck incision, for facelifts, 70
Necklift, 75–83
  background to, 75
  contraindications to, 76
  indications for, 75
  issues in, 82–83
  operative planning, 79
  operative technique, 79–82
  regional anesthesia for, 79
  patient information prior to, 76–77
  surgeon information prior to, 77–79
  variations in, 82
Nipple
  blood supply to, 27
  nerve supply to, 27
  "star gazing," 36
Nipple pedicle, variations of, 37
Nipple placement, defining, 36
Nose, deviated, 111

Obicularis oculi muscle, lateral, 71–72
Operative design
  in augmentation mammaplasty, 16
  in breast reduction/elevation, 28–29
  in facelift, 63–64
  in forehead lift, 88
Operative planning
  for abdominoplasty, 41
  for blepharoplasty, 53
  for necklift, 79
  for rhinoplasty, 102–103
Operative technique
  for abdominoplasty, 43–48
  for augmentation mammaplasty, 16–21
  for blepharoplasty, 54–56
  for breast reduction/elevation, 30–35
  for chemical peel, 117–118
  for collagen injections, 121
  for dermabrasion, 115
  for facelift, 64–68
  for forehead lift, 89–95
  for necklift, 79–82
  for rhinoplasty, 106–111
Orbicularis muscle hyperplasia, 56
Osteotomy methods, alternate, 111

Outfracture, in rhinoplasty, 112
Overgrafting, dermabrasion for, 114

Palpebral crease, upper, creation of, 57
Patient selection
  religious considerations in, 7–8
  screening process in
    additional, 6–7
    initial, 5–6
Pentobarbital (Nembutal), 11
Periareolar incision, for augmentation mammaplasty, 22
Pinocchio tip, nasal, 111
Plastic surgery, *see* Aesthetic surgery
Preauricular incision, for facelifts, 70
Principle of totality, 8
Pseudopalsy, of lower lip, 63

Reconstructive surgery, *see* Aesthetic surgery
Reduction/elevation, of breast, 25–38
Regional anesthesia, 16
  for blepharoplasty, 54
  for dermabrasion, 114
  for necklift, 79
  for rhinoplasty, 103–105
Religious considerations, in patient selection, 7–8
Rhinoplasty, 99–112
  background to, 99
  contraindications to, 100
  indications for, 99
  issues in, 112
  operative planning, 102–103
  operative technique, 106–111
  preoperative evaluation, 102–103
  preoperative marking, 103
  patient information prior to, 100–101
  regional anesthesia for, 103–105
  surgeon information prior to, 101
  variations in, 111–112
Rhytidectomy, *see* Facelift

Saddle nose deformity, 111
Scars, dermabrasion for, 113
Screening process, in patient selection, 5–7
Sedation
  for aesthetic surgery, 9–12
  choice of drugs, 11
  failure of, 11–12
  importance of, 9–10
  words as preoperative, 10
Skin/muscle flap, vs. skin flap, 57
"Star gazing nipple," 36
Subpectoral implantation, for augmentation mammaplasty, 22–23
Superficial muscular aponeurotic system (SMAS), 71–72

Suprabrow incision, for forehead lift, 96–97
Surgery, aesthetic, *see* Aesthetic surgery

Temple incision, for facelifts, 69–70
Temple lift, 95–96
Tip first/dorsum first, in rhinoplasty, 112
Tip projection, nasal, 111
Transfixion incision, in rhinoplasty, 112

Valium (diazepam), 11
  for facelift, 64
Valve interruption, in rhinoplasty, 112

Weir wedges, 111
Words, as preoperative sedation, 10
Wrinkles, circumoral, dermabrasion for, 113

Xylocaine, 16
  for blepharoplasty, 54
  for dermabrasion, 114
  for facelifts, 64
  for forehead lifts, 88
  for rhinoplasty, 104

Zyderm, 121